Racism and Race

The Use of Race in Medicine and Implications for Health Equity

UCSF Population Health and Health Equity

Proceedings of the Colloquia on Race in Medicine, March 24 - May 26, 2021

University of California
Medical Humanities Consortium
Department of Humanities and Social Sciences
UCSF (Box 0850)
490 Illinois Street, Floor 7
San Francisco, CA 94143-0850

ISBN: 978-1-7355423-4-8
DOI: 10.5072/FK2ZS2V40S

Designed by Virtuoso Press

University of California Medical Humanities Press

UC Medical Humanities Press publishes scholarship produced or reviewed under the auspices of the University of California Medical Humanities Consortium, a multi-campus collaborative of faculty, students, and trainees in the humanities, medicine, and health professions. Our series invites scholars from the humanities and health care professions to share narratives and analysis on health, healing, and the contexts of our beliefs and practices that impact biomedical inquiry.

General Editor

Brian Dolan, PhD, Professor, Department of Humanities and Social Sciences, University of California, San Francisco (UCSF)

Other Titles in this Series

Heart Murmurs: What Patients Teach Their Doctors
Edited by Sharon Dobie, MD (2014)

Humanitas: Readings in the Development of the Medical Humanities
Edited by Brian Dolan (2015)

Follow the Money: Funding Research in a Large Academic Health Center
Henry R. Bourne and Eric B. Vermillion (2016)

Soul Stories: Voices from the Margins
Josephine Ensign (2018)

Memory Lives On: Documenting the HIV/AIDS Epidemic
Edited by Polina Ilieva (2020)

---

www.UCMedicalHumanitiesPress.com

This series is made possible by the generous support of the Dean of the School of Medicine at UCSF, the UCSF Library, the California Digital Library, and a Multicampus Research Program Grant from the University of California Office of the President. Grant ID MR-15-328363.

Contents

Preface & Acknowledgments

During my time at the University of California, San Francisco (UCSF), I have had a number of rich, nuanced, and sometimes challenging discussions with colleagues and learners on the topic of racism and race, and more specifically how we use racial categories in our research and in the practice of medicine. I admire the deep commitment to health equity that guides so many on our campus, the shared goal we have of doing the right thing for our patients and ensuring the best for *all* of our patients. I have also been struck by the divergence of views on what the "right thing" is when it comes to the use of racial categories in medicine, even among deeply principled people committed to justice.

The insights I've gained from these discussions motivated this symposium on *Racism and Race: The Use of Race in Medicine and Implications for Health Equity*, hosted by the UCSF School of Medicine, in partnership with our sister Schools of Medicine at the University of California. In the process of planning and then hosting this event, several things have been clear to me: the critical, but often overlooked, need to understand the history and legacy of racism in medicine even as we proceed with our current work; the important insights that are gained from including diverse disciplinary perspectives, but are sometimes missed in our standard approaches to the teaching and practice of medicine; and the value of space for open and honest discussion, debate, and disagreement on a complex topic.

Academic medical centers are at their best when we cultivate this type of discourse that includes divergent views, values history and context, and moves from discussion to implications for the classroom, the clinic, and our scholarship. How we consider racial categories in medicine is critically important to our work as scholars and practitioners, as teachers and learners, but mostly our thoughtful and considered actions in this domain are important to the patients and communities we serve.

I am grateful to the UCSF School of Medicine for sponsoring this symposium. I am grateful to the many, many faculty, staff, and learners who participated in the planning and execution during the particularly difficult period of the COVID-19 pandemic; the people involved are named in their respective sections. I am appreciative of Dr. Brian Dolan for encouraging the creation of these proceedings and for shepherding the process and to UCSF PhD student Alice Guan for expert transcription of the sessions. And I am deeply indebted to Dr. Christine Dehlendorf and Stephanie Belger who carried the vision with me from beginning to end.

Kirsten Bibbins-Domingo, PhD, MD

Introductory Remarks

Kirsten Bibbins-Domingo, PhD, MD, UCSF

Good morning, and welcome to our series of discussions on the use of race in medicine, and the implications for health equity. I'm Kirsten Bibbins-Domingo, Professor and Chair of the Department of Epidemiology and Biostatistics at UCSF. I'm also Professor of Medicine, and the inaugural Vice Dean for Population Health and Health Equity in the UCSF School of Medicine. The Dean's office in the School has been pleased to host forums on topics that are timely and relevant to population health and health equity, and no topic is more timely or relevant than this one, especially for the practice and teaching of medicine that form the core of our mission in our medical schools. That is why we are pleased today to cohost this event with our fellow Medical Center campuses across the University of California.

I'd like to begin with this photo of our students. They are the inspiration for much of the discussion that we will have today. They have pushed us to have these types of discussions. They are the conscience of our campuses, and they force us to think about how we can live up to the ideals to which we aspire. This photo reminds me of the ways in which medicine and society are intertwined. Medicine reflects the larger societal discourse that we're having at this time, underscoring the urgency to dismantle structural racism and systemic oppression. But, in its practice and teaching, medicine also contributes to these larger social structures that we are addressing today.

Today, and throughout our subsequent meetings, we will explore a very specific slice of that larger conversation about racism and race in medicine: how we use racial categories in what we teach, in how we practice, and how we conduct research.

Our goal today is to lay the foundation for future discussions, and to understand the historical context of the use of race in medicine as well as current perspectives. We will then look at a series of case studies in the following meetings to explore this more deeply in its application to the work that we do on our campuses. We will conclude by delving deeper into our three mission areas, probing how lessons gleaned from the earlier sessions can inform how we should be teaching, practicing, and conducting research. In our final session we will have the opportunity to hold breakout groups to get down to the specifics of the implications of this for our own work.

The principles that have guided us in planning this series are two. The first is that we aspire to be an anti-racist institution. The second is that we are driven by health equity, the pursuit of health equity for our patients, for our communities, and for the populations that we serve. These are the principles that I am sure all of the speakers and organizers would espouse. It is in the application of these principles to the specific work that we do that there is complexity, that there is nuance, and there will be controversy. I think it's important for us as academic medical centers to embrace and tackle the nuance and complexity of these issues for our work. Zoom, I want to acknowledge is a wonderful platform that is allowing us to have this discussion with the more than 1000 of you that are registered for this session today. It is not always a platform that allows for the most nuanced of discussions, and so we acknowledge that there will be need for extending what we present here into other venues, and that we will continue to engage with these topics in the future.

We start with keynote presentations, followed by a moderated discussion with our keynote speakers. We will then have a second moderated discussion with a responder panel that includes colleagues from across the University of California system. We end with Q&A and closing comments.

I'm thankful for having had a fabulous steering committee with colleagues from across our UC campuses. The steering committee meetings were extraordinary and really had an enormous impact on how we structured these conversations, and I learned so much in each of meetings. I'm grateful to Dr. Christine Dehlendorf, Professor of Family and Community Medicine at UCSF, who is co-organizer of this event, and to Stephanie Belger, who is the Associate Dean for strategic initiatives in the UCSF School of Medicine, and who almost effortlessly got us to the point where we can have this complex series of discussions.

Race and Racism in Medicine: Historical and Theoretical Foundations

Dorothy Roberts, JD, FCPP, University of Pennsylvania

KIRSTEN BIBBINS-DOMINGO: I am thrilled that we have three really outstanding speakers and scholars to start us off on our discussions. First, we will hear from Professor Dorothy Roberts. She is the George A. Weiss University Professor of Law and Sociology at the University of Pennsylvania, Raymond Pace and Sadie Tanner Moselle Alexander Professor of Civil Rights, Professor of Africana Studies, and Director of the Penn program on Race, Science, and Society.

DOROTHY ROBERTS: Thank you, Kirsten, for that introduction and for the invitation to speak in this important session this morning. I've been asked to give a historical and theoretical foundation for our discussion of race and racism in medicine. And I do believe that understanding where current thinking about race in medicine originated can help us work toward being anti-racist in our future works.

To understand how race is used in medicine today, we need to trace current concepts of race and their relationship to racism all the way back to the very origins of the race concept, to the invention of the idea that human beings are naturally divided into distinguishable biological races. The belief in biological races whose bodies work differently originated in the scientific invention of race and the racial invention of modern science.

The expansion of the slave trade in the 1700s necessitated an expanding conceptual framework of race both to justify enslaving human beings and to govern a society based on forced human labor. At the end of the 17th century, many European theologians held that God created the races and made Europeans in his image. With the Enlightenment, the divine was no longer an acceptable basis for scientific evidence, so European scientists pointed to nature instead of God as the force that produced innate distinctions between races, but they basically imported this premodern creationism and racial mythology into modern science. Johann Blumenbach, for example, believed that some force of nature – and he borrowed this idea directly from Christian theology – had created five races: Caucasian, Malay, Mongolian, Native American and Ethiopian. He argued that they all descended from so called Caucasians.

Thomas Jefferson gives an example of this racial idea and how it was useful to excusing racial inequality. Race was invented to justify dispossessing indigenous people in the Americas and enslave African people and later to exclude them from the new nation, which was supposedly founded on the inalienable rights to liberty and equality. Of course, this posed a problem. How were you going to enslave people while supposedly creating a new nation founded on the opposite of slavery? Jefferson's writings show how the false belief in biological race was useful, because he could say that it *wasn't* because of violence or racism or power, it was because of the real distinctions nature made. This explained why it was okay to enslave people in a nation founded on liberty, just as the Catholic Church had used biological race as an excuse for enslaving Black people who converted to Christianity.

So, race is a system of made-up categories for governing people in an unequal society. Black people are defined as anyone with any African ancestry, regardless of the amount of variety of their non-African ancestors. Of course, we all have African ancestors, it just depends on what point in time you're going to start counting, which is made up as well. But white people have to be pure to qualify to be white. Well, that's because it was politically useful to white people to construct the categories that way in creating a society where many Black people could be enslaved, but only an exclusive group of white people could dominate them. We still use this political classification system today because it has been enforced since colonial times by legal definitions, court decisions, anti-miscegenation laws, and other Jim Crow laws—and extra-legal terror.

In the United States, doctors were essential to legitimizing the slavery system based on natural racial differences, rather than on racial violence and subordination. They promoted the racial concept of disease, that people of different races have different diseases, and experienced common diseases differently. In the 1850s, Southern physician Samuel Cartwright contended that Black people had lower lung capacity than white people and were therefore healthy only when enslaved and forced to work by whites. In his 1851 report on the *Diseases and Peculiarities of the Negro Race*, Cartwright described a list of diseases that he said were peculiar to Black people, all supposedly supporting his claim that enslavement was good for Black people's health. One of the most striking was his diagnosis of Drapetomania, a mental disorder that supposedly explained why some Black people ran away from plantations. Even after slavery ended, Cartwright's ideas that Black people have lower lung capacity stuck, and that's commonly believed today. Doctors adapted the racial concept of disease to argue that Black people bore a greater burden of disease because enslavement had kept at bay their natural propensities toward disease, and that their bodies now could not adapt to freedom.

The scientific belief in Black bodily difference also legitimated unethical experimentation on Black people, supposedly, to benefit their health.

So, when the human genome was mapped and the first draft of it was unveiled at a White House ceremony in 2000, everyone involved said, "Oh, well, it shows that there is no such thing as race at the genetic level." Bill Clinton emphasized that, in genetic terms, human beings are 99.9% the same. It would have been helpful if he also pointed out that the small amount of genetic difference does involve lots of genetic variation, but it can't be grouped by race.

So, many people thought, "Okay, now finally, we're going to get rid of this biological concept of race in medicine and biomedical research, and maybe even more broadly in American society." But instead, what happened was just the opposite. We saw a resurgence in interest in looking for race based genetic differences. And the definitions that originated in a false Christian theology that God created the races and then were taken up in the Enlightenment period to justify slavery, that nature created the races, now was turned into a new genetic or genomic definition that evolution created the races, with definitions like "races are population clusters based on genetic differences due to evolutionary pressure." But it's all basically the same idea: that nature, or some force of nature, whether God or just a spirit, or evolution, created races instead of what we know to be true—that race is an invented political categorization system to govern people and to specifically govern people in an unequal society.

So, when I began to see this resurgence of interest in looking for genetic differences between races, I wrote a book called *Fatal Invention: How Science, Politics and Big Business Recreate Race in the 21st Century*, and pointed out that race was being redefined as a genetic grouping. Again, the same basic definition from the 1600s, but now redefining it in terms of genetics. That genetics explains racial inequities, including inequities in health, and that this was seen as a basis for justifying race-specific biological remedies, including remedies supposedly for health inequities.

When the American Society of Human Genetics met in 2018, they had to confront the fact that white nationalists were using some geneticists' racial research to support their claims about innate racial differences. The society issued yet another statement, and there have been lots of these statements over the last half century or more – since the end of World War Two, really – in response to Nazi scientists using biological concepts of race. And we've seen statement after statement about the misuse of biological, more currently, genetic research involving race. But they made it seem as if there's only a problem with using biological concepts of race if you're a white nationalist. There remains lots of confusion within the field of genetics, within biomedical research and medical practice, about the use of race. I and three colleagues, Michael Yudell, Sarah Tishkoff, and Rob DeSalle, recently reiterated our appeal to the NIH that they confront the use of race in science and make efforts to end the confusion about when it's appropriate to use race, what race means, what are the implications of using race in in biomedical research.

There seems to be this persistent misunderstanding or failure to come to grips with the connection between biological concepts of race and racism. A natural division of human beings into races did not cause racism. Racism necessitated the invention of race, the human (not natural) classification of people into socially-constructed groupings that we call "races."

The false biological concept of race, and racial concept of disease, continue to misdiagnose health inequities. Take, for example, this research hypothesis from a 2007 study that appeared in a leading peer reviewed journal, the *American Journal of Obstetrics and Gynecology*: "Black race, independent of other factors, increases the risk of extreme preterm births, and its frequency of recurrence." "Black race, independent of other factors, increases risk." First of all, what is Black race? As I pointed out before, the definition in the United States of Black race is not the same, even the same kind of definition we give to white race. There are inconsistent ways of defining race, which you can only explain in political terms, and that definition varies across time. It varies across nations. It is completely determined by political imperatives at the current moment. And so, what do we mean by Black race? How do you identify, scientifically, people who have Black race and those who don't? How much African ancestry do you need to qualify? The way we generally think about it is *any* amount. And how can you possibly control for every factor other than this thing called Black race that might affect extreme premature birth? What's more, isn't it more plausible that factors other than some imagined innate Black race contribute to high rates of premature birth in Black communities in the United States? Wouldn't it be far more useful to study and address those factors, instead of leaving them out explicitly from a study?

These concepts are literally embedded in medical technologies. In routine lab results, the estimate for glomerular filtration rate for example, an important indicator of kidney function is listed as two different numbers – one for non-African Americans, and a higher healthier one for African Americans. In other words, eGFR automatically and categorically treats Black patients differently than all other human beings. Race based adjustments like this one are routine in diagnostic algorithms currently used in clinics and clinical research across the United States and approved a standard medical practice.

In addition, we know that Black people have been undertreated for pain. So another problem this exemplifies with race based medicine is that it promotes harmful stereotypes about racial bodily differences, making patients and research participants of color more vulnerable to mistreatment by healthcare professionals and researchers who believe these myths. It's long been documented that clinical staff undertreat Black patients for pain. Studies have shown that Black patients with painful long bone fractures and Black children suffering from appendicitis are far less likely than their white counterparts to get adequate pain treatment. A recent study of medical students and residents at University of Virginia medical school tied the undertreatment of Black patients' pain to absurd stereotypes about Black people's bodies, that Black people have thicker skin and less sensitive nerve endings than white people. The researchers found that a substantial number of white medical students and residents held these false beliefs about biological differences between Blacks and whites, and that these beliefs predicted racial bias in pain perception and treatment recommendation accuracy.

Although the COVID pandemic has impacted everyone in the nation, African Americans have borne the brunt of sickness. They've contracted and died from the virus at far higher rates than white Americans. Why? Dueling hypotheses about the answer go to the heart of our discussion today. Some scientists and politicians speculated that there must be something innately peculiar to Black people that made us more susceptible to illness and death. A better explanation is the conditions created by structural racism that put Black people at greater risk of disease and death. As the former president of the American Public Health Association, Dr. Camara Jones put it, "racism, not race, is a risk factor for dying of COVID-19." And I think that mantra is very helpful in general when we think about race in and racism in medicine. It's racism, not race, that is a risk factor.

The scientific challenge to biologically deterministic explanations for health inequities goes back at least a century. W.E.B. Du Bois contested the common wisdom in 1899 that newly emancipated Black people had poor health because their bodies were naturally ill prepared for freedom. In that tradition, there's mounting evidence that racial disparities and health are caused by structural racism. More and more studies at the intersection of the social and biological sciences are documenting the devastating impact of structural racism on Black people's health.

I think we can sum up the mechanisms uncovered by this research as embodying racism, the way racism gets under the skin to produce health inequities. Race isn't a biological category that naturally produces health disparities because of genetic difference. Race is a political category that has staggering biological consequences because of the impact of social inequality on people's health. This isn't a colorblind approach. It recognizes that race is a very real way our society categorizes people, and that this categorization shapes every aspect of our lives, including our health. That's precisely what the invention of race was designed to do. Pretending that race was created by some force of nature obscures reality.

A few years ago, I teamed up with Dr. Jonathan Metzl, the Director of the Center for Medicine, Health and Society at Vanderbilt University, to describe how racism has structured medical knowledge and practice, and to offer suggestions for ending it. Structural competency, a concept Dr. Metzl developed with Dr. Helena Hansen, who will be a panelist later today, describes an approach to medical training that emphasizes understanding how structural forces affect patients' health. In our article, we analyzed how racism in particular structures medical knowledge and practice and how healthcare professionals can work toward change. I think insights about structural competency and anti-racism in medicine apply as well to medical practice and research.

So, in the end, the best way to end health inequities is the best way to improve everyone's health: that is to work collectively to end structural racism and other inequities and towards a society that values every human being equally. A more equal and just society would be a healthier one. Thank you.

KIRSTEN BIBBINS-DOMINGO: Thank you very much. That was really terrific for setting the stage for us. I want to start with what you so nicely laid out: why are categories of race not biologically driven, and that racism has, in fact, created those categories. The study that you cite from the medical literature is a very familiar formulation of how we would normally do research, even disparities research: to say we've controlled for the other things. And now, we still find that black races are related to this. If we say that we don't want to be colorblind, but we want to understand disease burden that might be driven by racism, how do we capture racism in those types of studies? How should we be thinking of the sets of patients who have a greater burden of disease? We believe racism is the reason, but how should we capture that and measure that in order to explore it?

DOROTHY ROBERTS: I think the first point in designing studies is that the theory behind the study has to be that you are looking for the impact of racism on people's health. There may be a study where you're trying to determine the impact of some other aspect of social inequality, or you're trying to determine something apart from the impact of social inequality. There may be lots of research aims that you have. And the first thing is to be concerned about whether race is relevant to what you want to find out, and then how you define it.

I would say that race becomes relevant if you're looking for how racism affects people's health. So, the very first part of it is to be clear in the hypothesis, in the design, in the variables that you're using, that you're not basing it on a false idea of what race is. That's the most important thing. You know, I am not a biomedical researcher. And I think that we need to be innovative in ways that do include sociologists and legal scholars like me, along with biologists and others in figuring out how to design these studies. But I don't think we've done it well so far. The studies, I think, that are the best are the ones that have been looking at innovative ways of figuring out how racism gets embodied or gets under the skin, where their purpose is to study racism. And so, they're more careful about the fact that when they use Black, white, Latinx, Native American, etc., that they're using a socially constructed category. They don't pretend that it's some innate essence or it is something that's innate in the bodies of the people they're studying that are producing these outcomes. They're designing a study that's explicitly looking at how racism affects these people because of the social category that they're identified with. And so, being clear about the purpose of the study, and the meaning of the variables is an important start.

Just to take one aspect of what I've been saying: from that study, I pointed to Black race, there's no definition in the study of what the scientists meant by Black race, what the researchers meant by Black race. How are you identifying which participants belong in this group? If you are doing a study that claims that some innate factor puts the participants at risk, then how do you define who has that innate factor? In my opinion, it shouldn't be a social grouping that could include extremely different people.

I mean, if you just take the grouping Black, so Black race, who's in the Black race? It could be somebody who has one Black, great, great, great, great, great-grandmother, and everybody else is white, or Asian, or native. It could also be someone who just immigrated to the United States from Nigeria, whose ancestors were from Africa. So how could you put those two people in one study and say that they must have this innate factor you're looking for because we call them Black? That's just the most basic part of it. It's just the variables that you're using and defining them, let alone these deeper questions about how you design a study, who you collaborate with to make sure that you're capturing the actual meaning of race and the various ways that racism can affect the body.

I kind of pick on that study because the hypothesis was so clear, and so clearly wrong. But also to say independent of all other factors. So, are you really going to control for every social factor that could affect premature birth? I think you and I could sit here and we could think of 100 factors, and the study only controlled for a handful of factors. And it didn't control for the experience of racism. Does it control for the stress of racism? Does it control for the amount of years that someone lived in poverty? Does it control for environmental toxins in the neighborhood? Does it control for police presence in the neighborhood?

We could go on and on and on with all the ways that racism structures people's lives in America, and that would have to be taken into account in a study that claims to control for all factors independent of so-called Black race. So, those are some ideas about what we need to do and what we shouldn't do. One more thing is that it would be helpful for researchers who have a hypothesis like that to consult with people who are aware of how structural racism affects health, or even just aware of all the ways that structural racism affect our lives. They may not have thought explicitly about what's the impact on health, but they know about residential segregation. They know how that makes people living in certain neighborhoods vulnerable to all sorts of hazards that are bad for your health, that people living in other neighborhoods aren't vulnerable to, are not exposed to. And a biomedical researcher may not know that. It may be more likely that a sociologist would know that, and there has to be a collaboration. And one more thing is that in these collaborations, we need equality of respect for the knowledge that people of different disciplines have.

I can't tell you how many times people have said to me, "Well, you're not a doctor, you know, what do you have to say about this?" And I always respond, "Well, clearly, I know more about race and racism than you do. So I have a lot to say about this topic." But there is this idea that the only people who know about how racism or race affects health outcomes are people who are trained in biology, and sometimes specific parts of biology, when that only gives us a partial understanding, especially if we understand that biology isn't just genes. Biology involves—has to involve—the environment and social factors as well.

Making Precision Medicine Socially Precise

Esteban Gonzales Burchard, MD, MPH, UCSF

KIRSTEN BIBBINS-DOMINGO: Well, I thank you so much for kicking us off with that great keynote. I'd like to turn it over to Dr. Burchard who is Professor of Bioengineering and Therapeutic Sciences, a pulmonologist, and Professor of Medicine at UCSF. He is the founder and director of the Asthma Collaboratory, and the Center for Genes, Environment and Health.

ESTEBAN BURCHARD: Thank you. It's an honor and a privilege to be here. My name is Dr. Esteban Gonzalez Burchard. I'm a physician. I'm trained in pulmonary and critical care medicine, genetic epidemiology and epidemiology. So, here's the big debate that we use in medicine as of today. It's a national debate. And it's whether or not we should use race or ethnicity in clinical and biomedical research.

The camp has really been divided into two social constructs. One is race is a social construct. And then there are people who advocate that race has biological aspects. However, we here at UCSF recognize that it's an interaction, and that the social structure of race, which is a social structure, does influence biologic outcomes such as genetics and epigenetics. And this debate has been brought to the forefront, at least at UCSF.

America's Racial Awakening

Dear UCSF Health Community,

On October 14th, we will be changing our reporting of eGFR (estimated glomerular filtration rate) in Apex. We are making this change to Apex in part related to our recognition that there remain a number of inappropriate uses of race in medicine. Such uses can perpetuate the incorrect belief that race has a biological basis. Over the next several months, we will be evaluating the use of race in the setting of other diagnostic tests. In addition, UCSF will be examining the larger picture of race in medicine to better inform our work in ways that improve our understanding and recognition of differences among people that impact health but result from genetic and environmental factors (including racism and other social determinants) rather than race itself. I encourage you to attend a campus wide symposium series entitled "Race-Conscious Medicine: Controversies and New Frontiers" that is slated to begin in January to further explore this critically important set of issues.

Thank you,

Josh

Josh Adler, MD
Chief Clinical Officer, UCSF Health
Vice Dean, Clinical Affairs, UCSF School of Medicine

UCSF Health UCSF

This is an email that was publicly distributed by our chief clinical officer at UCSF, questioning whether or not we, as physicians who see patients, should use race in our clinical decision making. Now, this is not unique to UCSF. It is a discussion that has gone nationwide, and many hospitals have elected to categorically throw out race for things such as kidney disease, and lung disease. Now, before I go on, I want to tell you a little bit about who I am.

I'm a Mexican American. I'm born in California. My mother was born in California. This is her father, who's the second from the right, a farm worker in California. [Fig. 2] And when I took this picture, I didn't realize that it was superimposed on the New England Journal of Medicine, and that'll become relevant shortly. We come from a racially admixed family. These are my great grandparents, my great grandfather in the middle, his daughter on his left, my grandfather on the top right. And you can see that we're racially mixed. We're Native American. We're African, as you can see by the hair. We're European.

This is how I looked when I was in college. [Fig. 3] I was able to break out of life of poverty growing up in the Mission District of San Francisco with a single mother by becoming a nationally recognized wrestler in college. I was a two-time NCAA academic All American. This is how I looked when I started medical school. And when Professor Roberts talks about the social determinants of health, I want to remind her that I've experienced these. Now, I look very different now than I did when I was back from college.

But the two gentlemen on the left, Esteban and my colleague at the time, Rob Dodds, who's a neurosurgeon at Stanford, on our on our way to our first medical school exam, were pulled over by the Stanford police in 1990. [Fig. 4] We were late for our first medical school exam. It reminds me of what happened

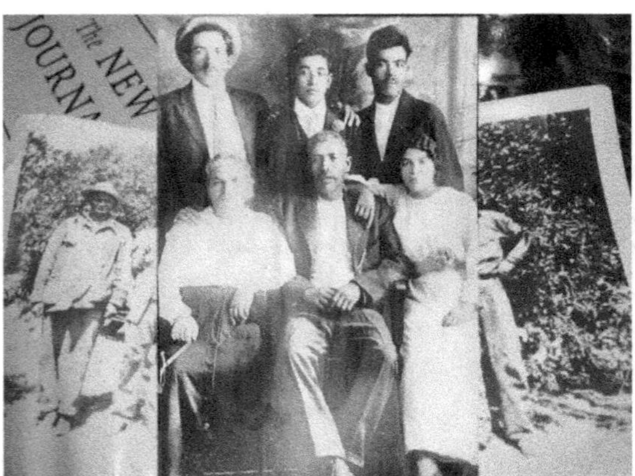

Fig. 2

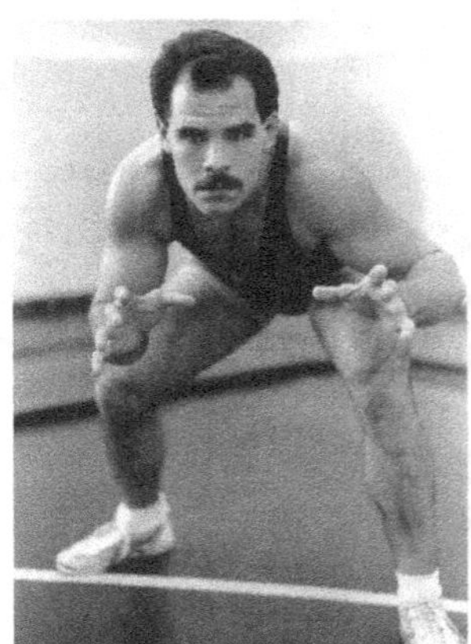

Fig. 3

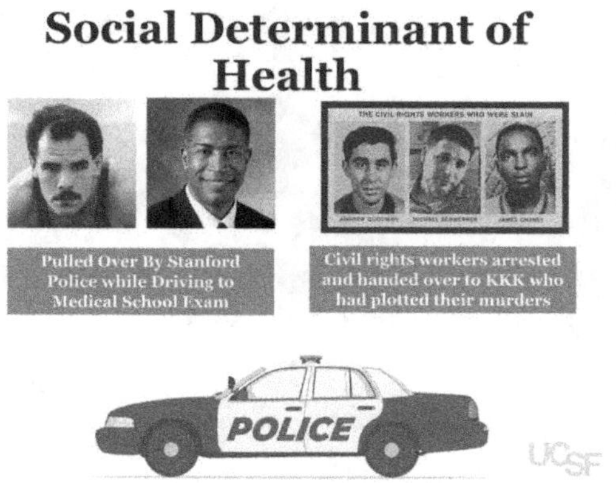
Social Determinant of Health
Pulled Over By Stanford Police while Driving to Medical School Exam
Civil rights workers arrested and handed over to KKK who had plotted their murders
POLICE
UCSF

Fig. 4

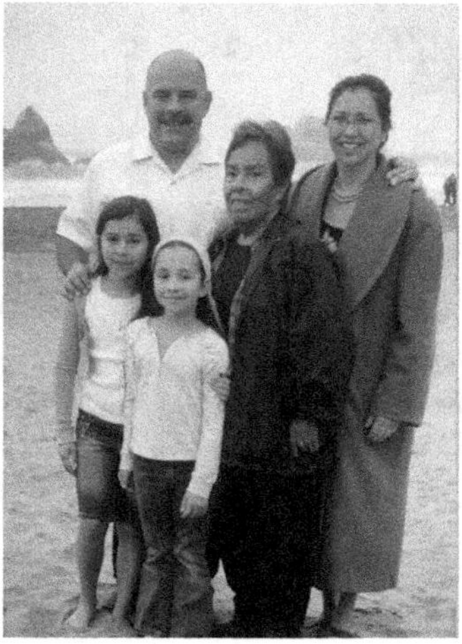

Fig. 5 (right)

in 1964, just 26 years earlier, when James Chaney, Andrew Goodman and Michael Schwerner, unfortunately, they were murdered, because the police turned them over to the KKK. But you cannot deny that when you're pulled over on the Stanford campus on the way to a medical school exam, that is going to have a negative impact on you.

This is my family before my mother passed away. You can see that she's very dark skin, and I'm very light skinned. So, that's always left me wondering about that Dr. Seuss book, are you my mother? Fortunately, I was able to get a sample of her saliva before she passed away and we went off to 23andMe and got tested. 23andMe is a private, soon to be public, company that came to fruition in 2004, along with other direct-to-consumer companies that marketed genetic ancestry testing, as well as disease testing, to consumers.

And you can see my mother's ancestry on the left, mine on the right. [Fig 6] You can see that my mother is more than half Native American, a substantial

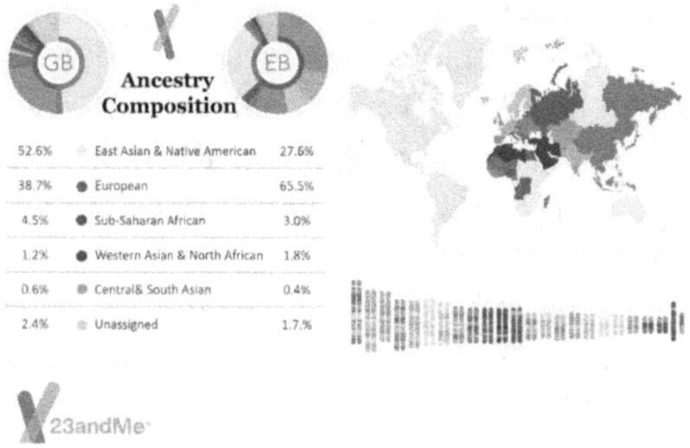

Fig. 6

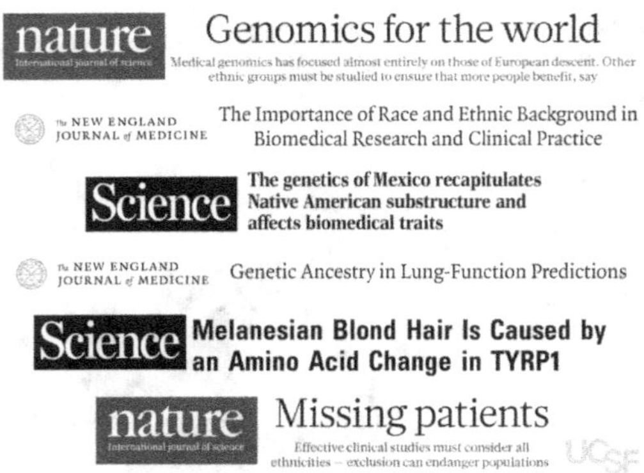
nature
International journal of science
Genomics for the world
Medical genomics has focused almost entirely on those of European descent. Other ethnic groups must be studied to ensure that more people benefit, say
The NEW ENGLAND JOURNAL of MEDICINE
The Importance of Race and Ethnic Background in Biomedical Research and Clinical Practice
Science
The genetics of Mexico recapitulates Native American substructure and affects biomedical traits
The NEW ENGLAND JOURNAL of MEDICINE
Genetic Ancestry in Lung-Function Predictions
Science
Melanesian Blond Hair Is Caused by an Amino Acid Change in TYRP1
nature
International journal of science
Missing patients
Effective clinical studies must consider all ethnicities — exclusion can endanger populations
UCSF

Fig. 7

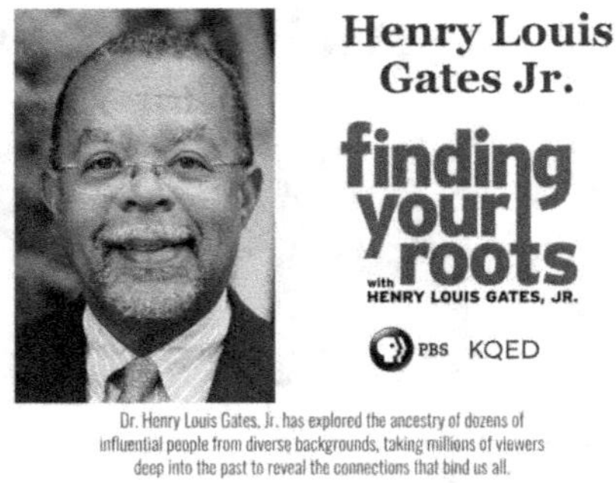
Henry Louis Gates Jr.
finding your roots
with HENRY LOUIS GATES, JR.
PBS KQED
Dr. Henry Louis Gates, Jr. has explored the ancestry of dozens of influential people from diverse backgrounds, taking millions of viewers deep into the past to reveal the connections that bind us all.

Fig. 8

amount of African. I have African ancestry. So according to Dorothy Roberts' definition, I am Black. But I've known this for a long time. And rather than put this on the shelf, we've made a career publishing, leveraging genetic ancestry in diverse populations to identify novel genes.

We've identified the blond hair gene in Melanesian populations, and that was published in *Science*. [Fig. 7] We identified the genetics of lung function in Mexicans, again published in *Science*. We had our first publication in the *New England Journal of Medicine* in 2003. And while I thought that most people didn't care, people like Henry Louis Gates, who are well established in academic circles, were off to the markets to make a significant amount of money touting the use of race and finding your roots, and everybody seems to be okay with that. [Fig. 8]

Now, at the same time, I was contacted by David Duke in 2003, right after our *New England Journal* paper and said, "Man, you are right on." And for those of you that don't know, by night, he's a Klansman. By day, he's an everyday voter. He's a politician, a member of the Parent Teacher Association, and a board member. My point in bringing this up is that he's still swimming amongst us. And what I want to bring up is that here is where we need social oversight, ethical oversight of anything we do with respect to genetics and medicine.

Now, as I said, I'm a specialist in lung disease. And at an early age, I was interested in asthma, mostly because it's the most common chronic disease of children. But mostly because of this: asthma is the one disease that has the

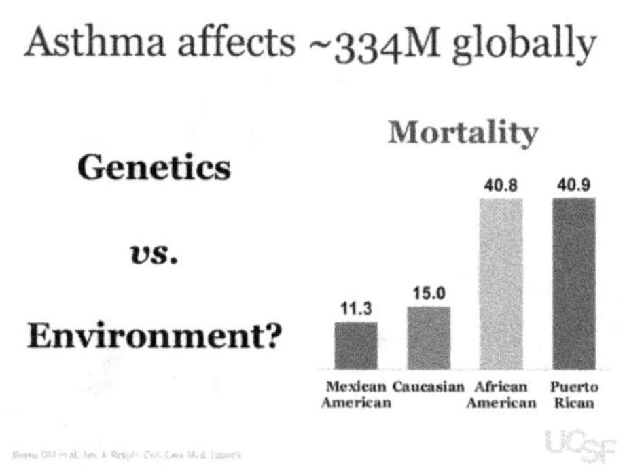

Fig. 9

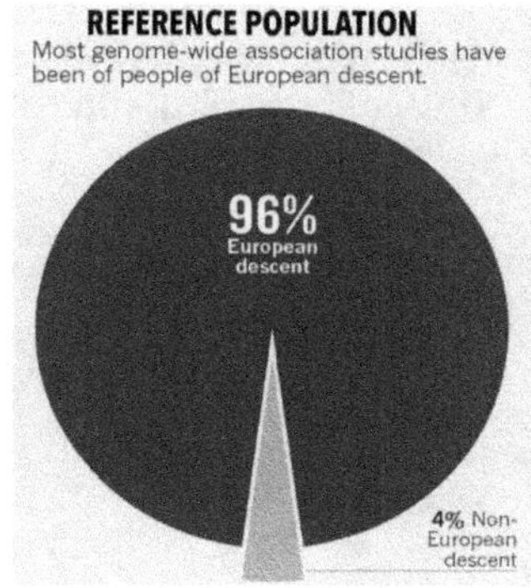

Fig. 10

most significant racial disparities in the world. Asthma prevalence, morbidity and mortality are highest in Puerto Rican populations and African American populations, and lowest in Mexican populations.

Despite that, over 95% of NIH research over the last 25 years has focused on white populations. So, my colleagues Carlos Bustamante and Francesco de la Vega did a systematic survey of all modern genetic studies in the United States, published up until 2009. We found that 96% were done in populations of European origin. Europeans make up less than 12% of the world population, yet they derive all modern benefits from the human genome project. So essentially, the Human Genome Project was the European Genome Project. Well, that's how we started off.

We created a study recruiting minority children throughout the United States. And like Professor Robert said, we brought in social epidemiologists that were experts at measuring race and racism, that are expert in measuring socioeconomic status, that were expert in measuring air pollution. And we brought in geneticists who can measure genetic ancestry. We recruited children from all over the United States, including Puerto Rico and Mexico to capitalize on the variation and diversity of air pollution and socioeconomic status and ancestry. [Fig. 11]

And today, we recruited over 11,000 minority participants and we're going strong. We have the largest study of minority children in the United States. [Fig. 12] And to do this correctly, we collected a variety of measures, including genetic factors, clinical factors, exposure history, diets and behaviors, perceived discrimination, socioeconomic status, and geocoded measures of air pollution. We used this information to differentiate individuals that were healthy from those that had asthma. And then, among those that had asthma, we used it to identify the different flavors of asthma because we know that peripheral blood cell counts differ by race and ethnicity. And it is those peripheral blood

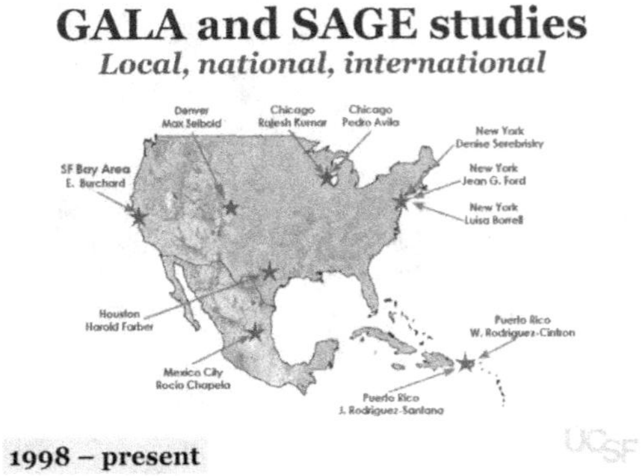

Fig. 11

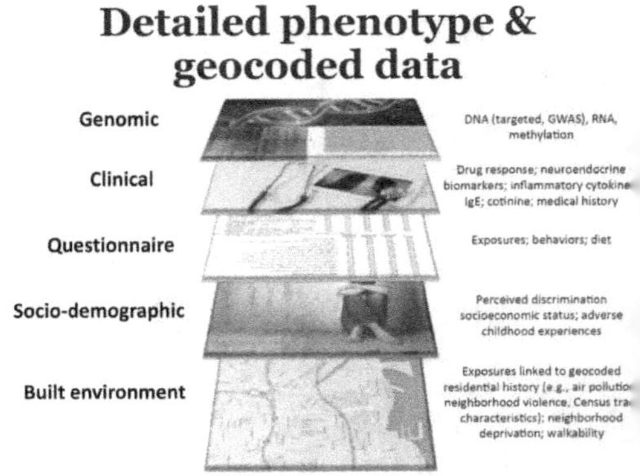

Fig. 12

cell counts that are used to treat patients. So, we demonstrated that African Americans and Puerto Rican patients do not derive the same benefit from modern asthma therapies called biologics than their white counterparts simply because of their blood cell count. It has nothing to do with their skin. It has everything to do with the peripheral white blood cell count.

Now, Professor Roberts had said that we are all from Africa and those dates can be disputed. But that's not true. We can actually pinpoint, with carbon dating, when people left Africa. People left Africa to go to Europe, to Asia, all around the world.

So, the contemporary world population is a subset of Africa. Africa has the most genetic diversity in the world. Every other population is a subset. Along the way, the new populations develop their own genetic variants that are private to Native Americans, private to Asians, and those genetic variants lead to differences in drug response and risk of disease. Now, a new event has happened in the last 500 years, and you know this event well. Christopher

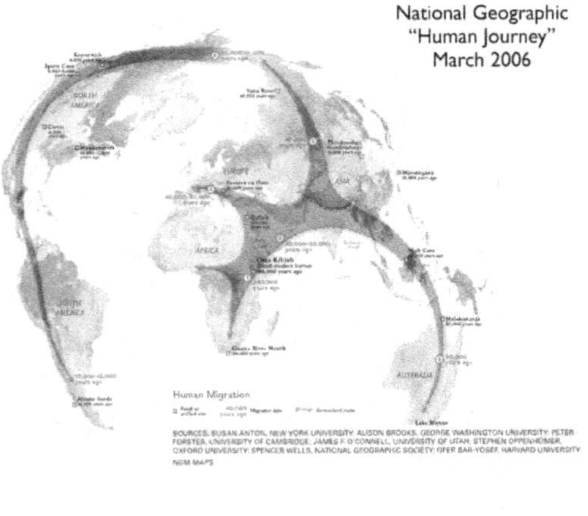

Fig. 13

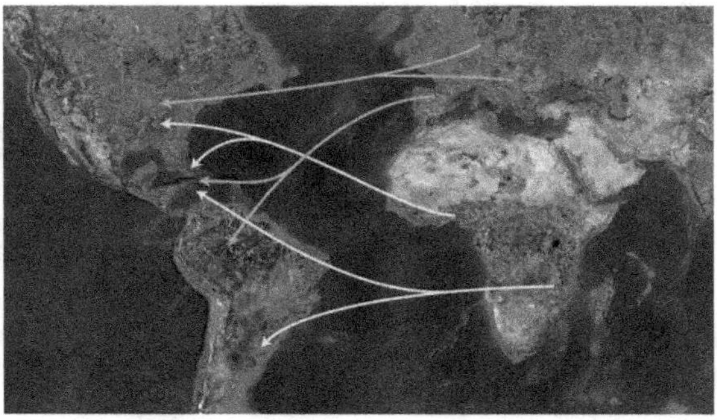

Fig. 14

Ancestry of Latinos & African Americans

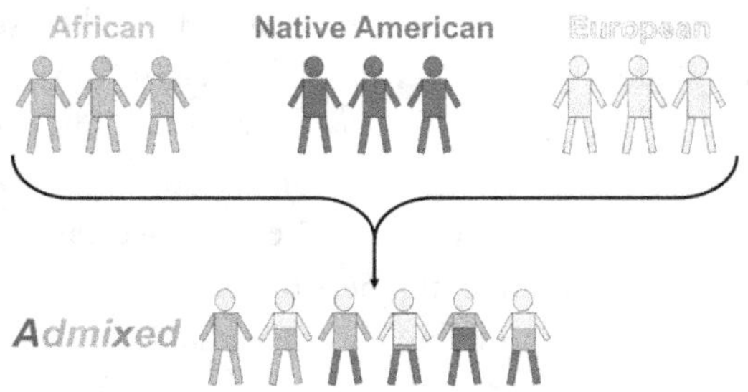

Fig. 15

Columbus came to the new world. He started the slave trade. Native Americans were already here in the new world, so there's a massive collision of three ancestral populations beginning in 1492. And the three populations are African, Native American, and European. [Figs. 14 and 15]

The contemporary population is what we call admixed, and that's what I try to show with the stick figures here with different proportions of colors, representing different proportions of genetic ancestry. So, like I said, I'm 27%, Native American, 6%, African, the rest is European. Now, this is all well and good, but does it have clinical relevance?

I am a physician. I'm a physician scientist, and I only care whether or not our work has meaningful clinical relevance. So, Professor Roberts had suggested that lung function was used inappropriately to justify slavery. Now, the spirometer was not developed to reinforce slavery. It was developed to measure lung function, and we use it every day worldwide in medicine to measure lung function.

And here's a little picture of little Juanito, who has asthma. [Fig. 16] He has a nose clip. He's breathing into the machine. On the top we have exhalation, on the bottom we have inspiration. The dashed line is before an administration of an asthma bronchodilator, and the solid line is after administration of the

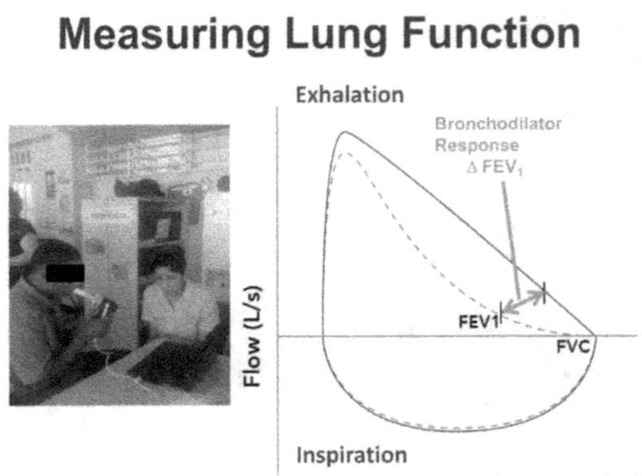

Fig. 16

drug bronchodilator. Now, we know that lung function is determined by sex. We know it's determined by age. We know it's determined by height. But what do we do in a diverse country like America in which over 50% of children are minorities, and over 36% of the population are African or Latino?

Well, when I arrived at UCSF in 1998, we used a white reference equation for everybody, just like the people who I'm debating here today are arguing for. And instead of having an African American reference equation, we just took the white equation and racially adjusted it by 15% lower for blacks, 8% lower for Asians.

Now, this is what we call race correction. [Fig. 17] Fortunately, the Center for Disease Control, recognized that there's diversity in the United States. And they started what was called the NHANES study, National Health examination and Nutrition Examination Survey, in which they set out mobile vans all over the country.

And you can see this diagram on the bottom, there's a reception area, there's a urine collection station, there's a breathing station, there's a dietary station, blood pressure, everything. [Fig. 18] And they did this, they standardized it.

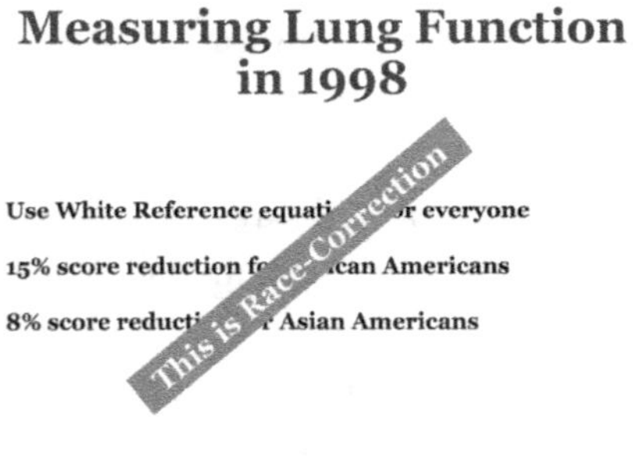

Fig. 17

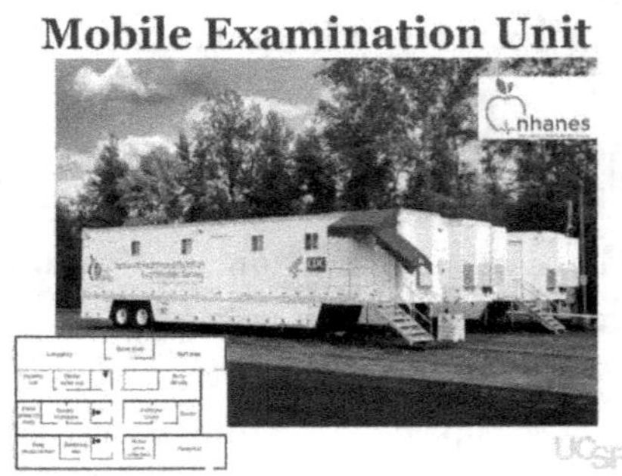

Fig. 18

Race/ethnicity & Lung Function

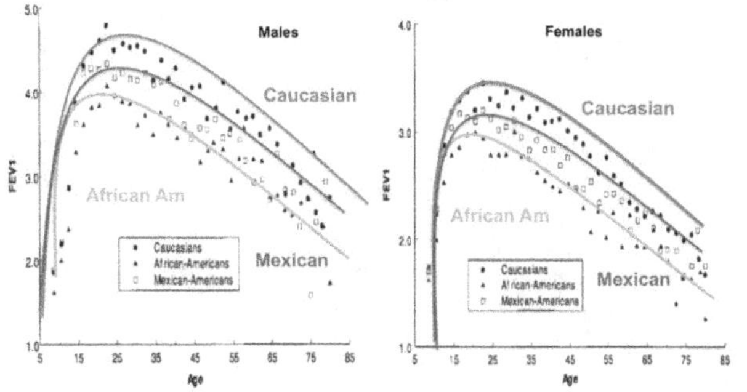

Figure 1. Mean FEV_1 versus age (2-yr increments) for male subjects.

Adapted from NHANES data - Hankinson JL et al. AJRCCM 1999

Figure 2. Mean FEV_1 versus age (2-yr increments) for female subjects.

Fig. 19

First, they went out and got all whites – you could only participate if you're healthy and white. They did all the measurements. They did the same thing for Mexicans – you can only participate if you're healthy, and self-identified as Mexican. Then they did this for African Americans, same thing. They measured lung function on everybody, kidney function on everybody. And they came up with normal distributions of what we consider to be healthy.

This slides a little complex. [Fig. 19] I'll walk you through it. On the x axis here, I have age going from five to 85. I have males on the left, females on the right. On the y axis, I have a lung function – the higher you are, the better. And what you see is, there are three different normal prediction standards – one for African, one for Mexicans, and one for Caucasians. And that's because when Little Johnny comes into the clinic, you want to make sure that you're comparing apples to apples. So if I tell you, Johnny is at the 70th percentile for height, you intuitively know that Johnny is taller than 70% of people his age, gender, and race and shorter than 30% of the population. Well, that's what we do in medicine. If you're African American, we want to compare you to African Americans. If you're Mexican, you want to compare you to Mexicans. If you're white, we want to compare you to whites. You'll notice that there are no Asian equations. There are no Southeast Asian equations. So those populations get compared to being white. Now, this is not race correction. Let me be very clear for the record. It is not race correction. It is not race adjustment. It is a race stratified analysis.

I had a firefighter who was African American, who had an on-the-job injury and came into my clinic. He obviously wanted to get disability benefits. The insurance companies inherently didn't want to pay, so they sent it to me as

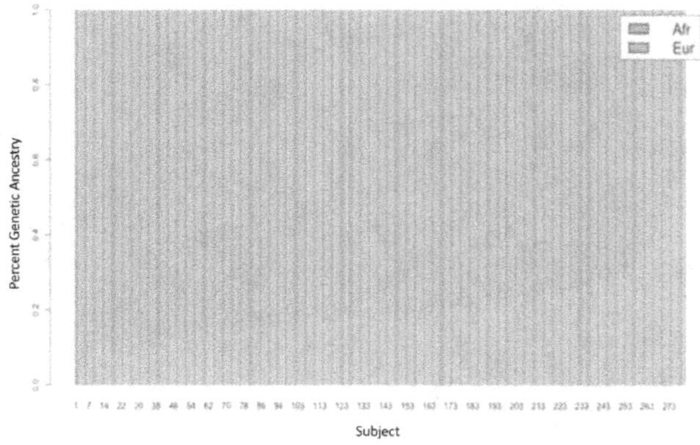

Intra-racial variability in ancestry

Fig. 20

an independent third-party physician. I knew about 23andMe. I knew growing up that I was racially mixed. I knew that this individual was racially mixed.

And here is a graphic display of ancestral proportions of 274 individuals, green being European ancestry, orange being African ancestry, every line represented an individual. [Fig. 20] So, President Obama would sit over here, way to the right. So, the question that you have to ask yourself, and I had to ask is, even though the clerk that took in his intake information called him African American when he got to my clinic, since I'm from the hood, I was able to code switch and say, "Hey, man, are you a brother? Or what?" And he goes, "Yeah, I'm half." And so that really began my journey, my scientific journey. Should we use self-identified race versus genetic ancestry? And so my colleagues and I studied seven independent, healthy cohorts of African American adults and children, and used genetic ancestry.

Ancestry & lung function (FEV_1)

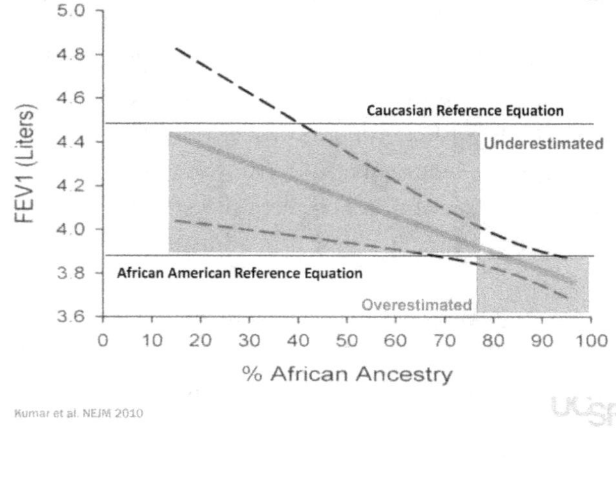

Fig. 21

This slide is complex. [Fig. 21] I'll walk you through it. On the *x* axis, we have increasing amounts of African ancestry. On the *y* axis, we have lung function – the higher you are, the better. And what you can see is that there's an interaction. And what we found is that when we compared our patient to the average reference equation for African Americans versus whites, we got different results. And essentially, depending upon an individual's genetic ancestry, if they were over 78% African ancestry, we overestimated their disease. If my patient was 50% African ancestry, we would underestimate their disease. Now, this again, is not race corrected. This is in African Americans only, who are healthy adults and children.

So, now that we prove this and we publish this in the *New England Journal*, we publish the same results for Mexicans in the journal *Science*. Pretty good for the son of farmworkers. The questions that the epidemiologist will ask or the social epidemiologists, are: do social ecological factors mediate or confound the relationship between genetic ancestry and lung function? In plain English, are our associations with genetic ancestry just a reflection of being born in a poor environment that has high air pollution, that has high amounts of racial discrimination? Is this the summation of all their life experiences? Since we have the largest study of minority children in the United States with the most comprehensive data, we were able to ask that question. [Fig. 22]

We studied 5500 Latino children from all over the United States and asked: What is the biggest driver of lung function? Is a genetic ancestry? Is it social environmental exposures, like secondhand smoke, air pollution, *in utero* smoking, number of siblings? Or is it socioeconomic factors: discrimination, acculturation, insurance. And what Maria Pino Yanes and my postdoc, Neeta Thakur, did with the help of Maria, who's a geneticist, they were able to demonstrate that the strongest predictor was genetic ancestry, even after adjusting for the confounders that we knew we could measure. Now, there's no perfect study, and we're never going to be able to adjust for all potential

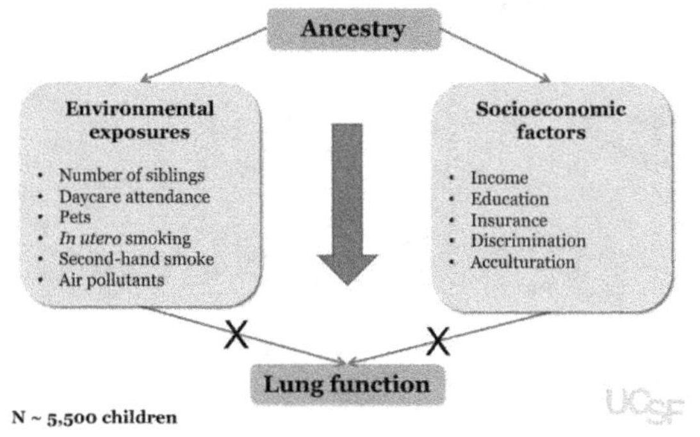

Fig. 22

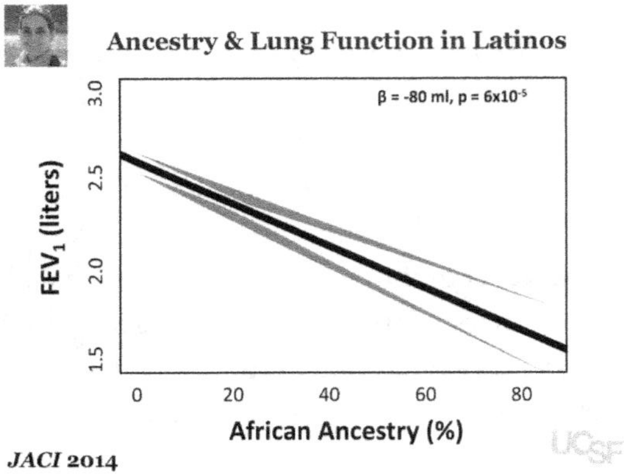

Fig. 23

confounders. But this is the most comprehensive study today on this topic.

What Maria went on and demonstrate is, amongst 5500 Latino children with and without asthma, African ancestry is associated with lower lung function. [Fig. 23] Now, what happens when we have discrepancies? What happens when we have disease misclassification? In the *New England Journal* paper, we demonstrated that there's an error rate of as much as 15%. How many of you would like a clinical exam, whether it be a tumor biopsy, etc., that had an error rate of 15%? In the *Science* paper, we demonstrated that there's an error rate of 10%. Well, when you have disease and classification, it leads to inappropriate referrals, inappropriate test, and it has significant clinical implications including disability rating, transplant referrals. Remember, the comedian, Martin, he died on a lung transplant list. If he were diagnosed earlier, he might have gone on the lung transplant list. It has implications for workers comp, and reimbursement for rehabilitation.

Now, here's a warning for us all. [Fig. 24] This is a paper published last week by UCSF Dr. Yulin Hswen, and this highlights the danger of the bully pulpit. Untrained popular personalities can have adverse consequences. Dr.

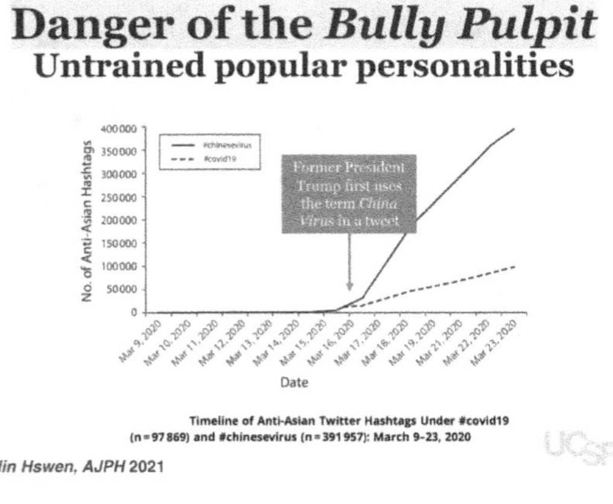

Fig. 24

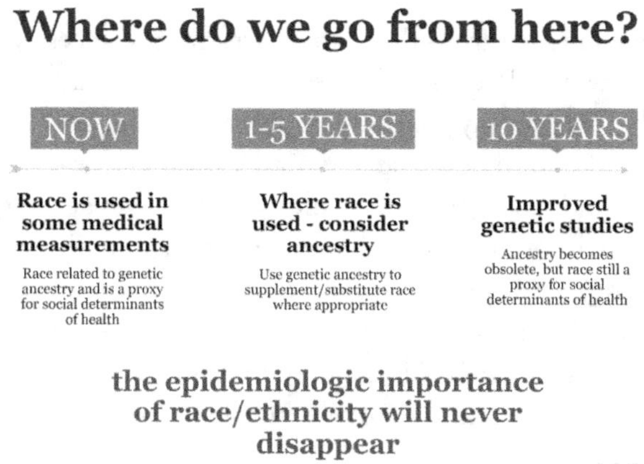
Where do we go from here?
NOW
1-5 YEARS
10 YEARS
Race is used in some medical measurements
Race related to genetic ancestry and is a proxy for social determinants of health
Where race is used - consider ancestry
Use genetic ancestry to supplement/substitute race where appropriate
Improved genetic studies
Ancestry becomes obsolete, but race still a proxy for social determinants of health
the epidemiologic importance of race/ethnicity will never disappear

Fig. 25

Hswen looked at the number of anti-Asian hashtags from March 16, 2020, to the rise in hate. And what this shows is that people who are untrained but very popular, who venture into fields that they know nothing about can have dangerous implications and consequences. And that's why we need to be careful. The consequences of throwing out race and ethnicity is like throwing out the baby with the bathwater. If we throw out race and ethnicity, we will default to the dominant population, which as of today, and probably for the next several decades, is going to be European origin. So, when someone says, "let's throw out race from GFR," they're saying, "Let's use the white equation for everyone." We need to have a clinical and scientific alternative before we carte blanche throw out race and ethnicity. And again, we have dangerous consequences for not educating ourselves before speaking and publishing.

So, where do we go from here? [Fig. 25] As of today, race is used in some medical measurements. It is used for lung disease, it is used for heart disease, it is used for kidney disease. It's used almost every measure that is known to medicine. Where are we going?

Genetic ancestry has been around since 2000, 21 years ago. The human genome project started 30 years ago, yet we as physicians and scientists have yet to include it into medical measures, such as lung function. To the best of my knowledge, we were the first to do it in 2005. We did it again in 2010. We do it again in 2014. And it's rearing its ugly head in 2021. Where are we going in the future? We predict that ancestry will become obsolete, and that race will still be a valuable proxy for social determinants of health. But I contend, and we recently published this in the *New England Journal* on the day of the insurrection, January 6, that the epidemiologic importance of race and ethnicity will never, ever disappear. It is a valuable construct that captures social determinants of health throughout your life. The takeaways that I would like you to get from this is that race, genetic ancestry and medicine are tightly intertwined. Race specific measures are not the same as race corrected measures. What we can say can have dangerous consequences. And that's a message, a reminder for myself and a reminder for my colleagues who are speaking today. The epidemiologic importance of race will never go away. Throwing race away without consideration is not an answer. We threw away race for kidney function and we told people to measure body mass. I can guarantee you that no physician is trained in how to measure body mass.

I'm going to end it there. But I want to thank many people from my close-knit team. I want to thank my mentor Neil Risch. I want to thank the Center for Genes, Environments and Health. My partners in crime, Elad Ziv, Jennifer Elhawary, Luisa Borrell, Noah Zaitlen, my whole entire lab, and the Sandler Foundation who helped me through the darkest days when the NIH wouldn't fund me. I went 0 in 11 at the NIH, despite having papers in the *New England Journal* and *Science*. And then I want to thank all my collaborators. I'm going to end it there, but I'll be happy to take any questions now. Thank you very much for the opportunity to speak.

KIRSTEN BIBBINS-DOMINGO: Thank you so much, Dr. Burchard. So, help us to understand, you've highlighted the importance of ancestry for an understanding and genetic variation for making these types of discoveries. But help us to understand a little bit more about this methodology. If, as you accept, that racism and socially constructed factors determine these racial categories, how do we ever completely disentangle when you map these genetic markers onto ancestral continents? The forces that are actually *social* from the ones that are actually *genetic*? Given that you are starting with self-identified race, and then clustering into these ancestral contexts, how do we really know that those are, in fact, genetic differences, as opposed to the cluster of social factors that that cluster with racism?

ESTEBAN BURCHARD: Well, that's actually a very important question. And I have two things to say. First of all, as of today, 2021, there's gross under representation of African, Indigenous, and people of color included in modern genetic studies. Things like H3Africa are making a dent. We need to have more studies like that.

There are environmental factors that shape genes. For example, sickle cell. The APOL1 L gene that is common in West Africa, relatively absent in East Africa, but because the United States has been largely populated with slaves from West Africa, they have a gene that has a protection from a parasite, and that's why it's been allowed to stay in the population. But it's a significant risk factor for the development of early stage kidney disease. So that's an example where there's a gene environment interaction.

Now, what happened in Ferguson and Michael Brown has nothing to do with genetics. That's purely social. If I told you as an insurance agent, what is the likelihood of an individual dying in Ferguson, Missouri? The first cut off would be is it male or female? The second cut off would be, Black or white? And then, it'll be your zip code and your GPA. So insurance actuaries use these proxies all the time, for determining risk. That has nothing to do with biology.

With regard to other studies, like the lung function one, as of today, it's an empiric question. We need to do the work. What is more important? Is it genetic? Is it social? Is it environmental? Or is it a combination of the two? If it is social and environmental, how do we weigh it? How do we weigh me being pulled over on my first day of medical school? How do we weigh that? How do we get internalized? You know, those experiences getting under our skin. And contrary to what Professor Roberts has said, epigenetic factors are inherited. They're passed down from one generation to another generation. It's been proven in Holocaust survivors. Epigenetics is inherited, and the perfect example that we have where we, as physicians, interfere with epigenetics every day, is pregnancy. We get pregnant mothers folate to change their genes to prevent spina bifida. That's an environmental intervention that causes epigenetic changes that are inherited by the child. So it's complex, Kirsten. It is complex, and Professor Roberts had it correct. We do need multi-disciplinary teams to help address this.

KIRSTEN BIBBINS-DOMINGO: Great. All right. Well, I want us to leave time for our last speaker and then invite everybody back for the panel. So please, let me invite Dr. Jones.

Historical and Current Perspectives on Race and Racism in Medicine and Implications for Health Equity

David S. Jones, MD, PhD, Harvard University

KIRSTEN BIBBINS-DOMINGO: Dr. David Jones is a Harvard College Professor, A. Bernard Ackerman Professor of the Culture of Medicine, Faculty of Arts and Sciences and Faculty of Medicine, and Professor of Epidemiology at the Harvard T.H. Chan School of Public Health.

DAVID JONES: Well, thank you for the invitation to participate in this terrific series of events that UCSF has launched. My predecessors have set a high standard. My remarks, as you will see, are more closely aligned with what Dorothy Roberts said. I'll try to compliment and not duplicate what she has already told us. And I'm certainly grateful that zoom will spare me from getting pulled into a wrestling match with Esteban, which he would clearly win. While I cannot claim a diverse African, indigenous, or European ancestry, and while I cannot claim to have been raised in the hood, I can say that I have educated myself before speaking and publishing, and I don't think any of us appreciate the comparison to Donald Trump in this context.

Many events over the past year have triggered an unprecedented reckoning with racism. [Fig. 1] Many within medicine acknowledge that we face multifaceted problems, from the structural racism in society that leads to health inequities, to the systemic racism within medicine that leads to disparate treatment of people of color, whether patients, medical students, physicians, or faculty.

Many institutions, including Harvard Medical School and UCSF have

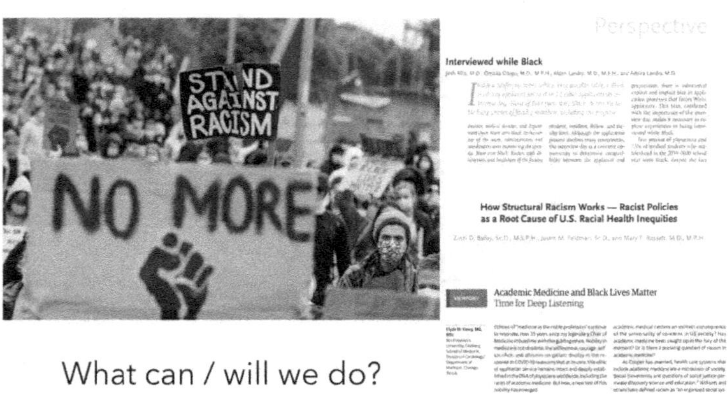

Fig. 1

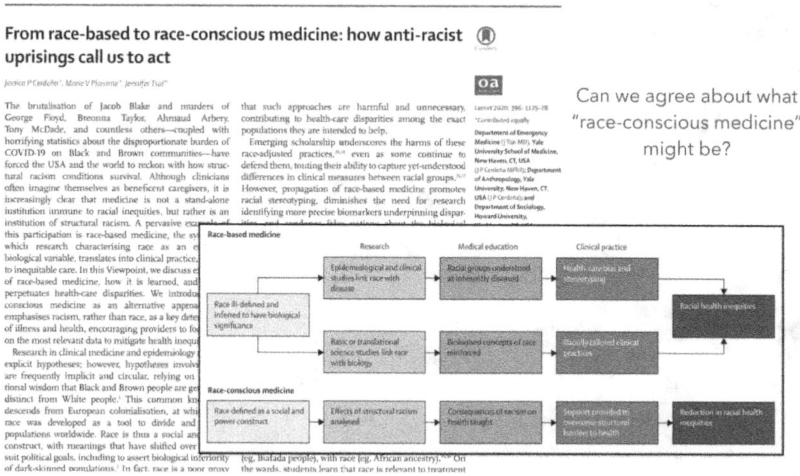

Fig. 2

committed themselves to antiracism. One challenge is that we don't yet know what that involves. One examples of this is the debate about the use of race in medical theory and practice.

Should we provide different care to people of different races and ethnicities because of their race and ethnicity? Many people say yes. They see race-based medicine as an evidence-based way to contribute to efforts to solve health inequities. Others see race-based medicine as the opposite, as neither scientific nor evidence-based, as just another form of bias that can accentuate inequities. Such practices also perpetuate the pernicious idea that race is a biologically meaningful category.

Critics of the use of race in medicine are often accused of calling for race-blind medicine. I don't know anyone who has done that. [Fig. 2] Protagonists on both sides of the debate actually support race-conscious medicine. But what is the best way for medicine to be race conscious?

In the short time I have, I will describe one area of debate: the role of race in diagnostic testing and treatment guidelines. Since subsequent sessions will drill into the details of these debates, I will focus instead on the fundamental questions at stake in these debates.

Over the past century, physicians have operationalized race in many ways in medicine. They have produced treatment guidelines and recommend adjusting treatment according to a patient's race or ethnicity. [Fig. 3] They have developed diagnostic tests and calculators that return different results based on a patient's race. Over the past several years, a few of these have come to national attention, especially tests to estimate the kidney function.

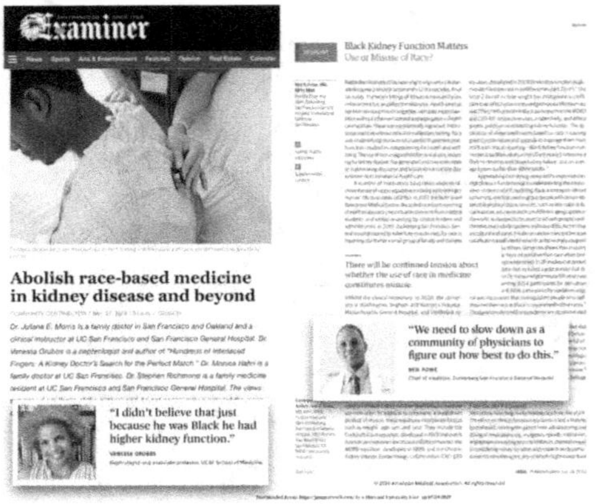

Fig. 3

Last June two of my former students and I published a review of race correction. We described 13 tools drawn from across many medical specialties. While there is evidence for each, it is often quite weak. Implementation of the tools also leaves much to be desired: many rely on a dichotomous variable of black or nonblack. We feared that these tools, if used as directed, could actually exacerbate health disparities, not alleviate them. [Fig. 4, below]

Our article, appearing in the aftermath of George Floyd's death and the Black Lives Matter protests, amplified the debated that had begun around eGFR. Race correction has become a major topic of discussion over the past year. Tensions around the issue were further inflamed by allegations that the NFL uses race correction of neuropsychological tests to deny settlements to retired black players.

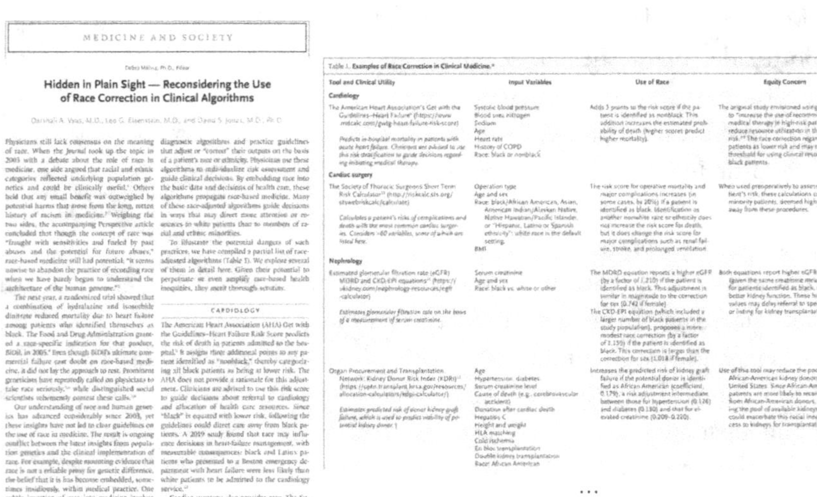

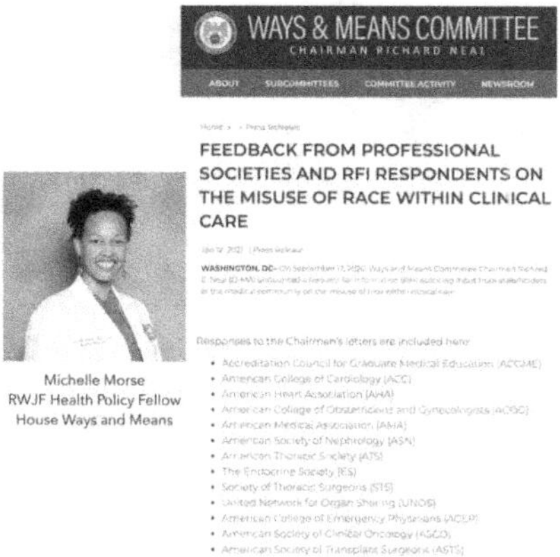

Fig. 5

This all caught the attention of Congress, in part because of the work of my colleague Michelle Morse. [Fig. 5] The House Ways and Means committee sent letters to many medical societies asking for an explanation of how they use race. AHRQ has now done something similar. In January Ways and Means posted the responses, a fascinating and complex set of readings.

Meanwhile, researchers have continued to publish many new analyses that highlight the misuse of race in medical school curricula or defend the use of race in health care. What should we make of all this?

First, we all need to be extremely careful in our scholarship. Race is both scientifically complex and emotionally charged. Many authors and readers have very strong feelings. Anyone who engages has a special obligation to be fastidious in their work. Unfortunately, it remains relatively easy to find mistakes by smart and well-intentioned researchers.

One article published in February falsely claimed that a combination of hydralazine and isosorbide dinitrate had been "repeatedly shown to be more effective for heart failure outcomes in Black patients than White patients." That simply isn't true. Cardiologists often assert that South Asians are responsible for 60% of all cases of cardiovascular disease worldwide. That can't possibly be true. Several groups have claimed that my June article had errors, misrepresentations, or understandings—though they haven't identified what those might be. We all need to do our best to make positive contributions to the debates.

Second, I am increasingly frustrated by an asymmetry that exists in medical thinking. Protagonists in the debates have demanded that critics proceed with great caution before ending any practice of race correction, for instance modeling what effects the changes might have. No one, however, proceeded with great caution when race correction was introduced. I haven't

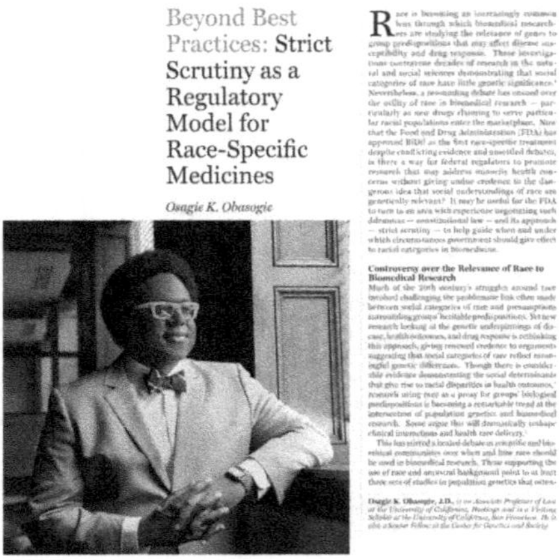

Beyond Best Practices: Strict Scrutiny as a Regulatory Model for Race-Specific Medicines

Osagie K. Obasogie

Controversy over the Relevance of Race to Biomedical Research

Fig. 6

done detailed research, but as best as I can tell researchers detected a race signal in data, offered a tool to address that, and won consensus to implement the change. This was often done without a rationale for the race correction, and without modeling how patients would be affected.

Osagie Obasogie, now on the faculty at Berkeley, has shown how courts have generally used a standard of "strict scrutiny" when policies or practices take race into consideration. [Fig. 6] Such scrutiny is being demanded before race correction is ended even though it was not used when race correction was implemented. I think that this asymmetry reflects a widespread assumption that race is real and should be acted on.

This raises my third concern, about the nature of race. This involves two distinct problems. The first is a question of taxonomy: is it meaningful to divide the human species into subspecies or races? Plato famously demanded that our categories "carve nature at the joints." Do race categories do that?

For several centuries, scholars in European intellectual traditions have seen race as a legitimate category—a natural kind—either because they reflected distinct acts of divine creation, or because they reflect divergent evolution of geographically distinct populations. In either sense, people assume that race correlates with ancestry, and that different ancestries are associated with distinct genetic variations.

There certainly is evidence for this. Geneticists have shown links between genetics and geography in many ways. For instance, if you careful select a population of Europeans, you can show fine-grained correlations between geography, ancestry, and genetics.

But how often are these race, ethnic, or ancestral categories—and their associated genetic variants—medically meaningful? This is the fundamental

The Ancient Question: are we similar or different?

> Hath not
> a Jew eyes? Hath not a Jew hands, organs, dimensions,
> senses, affections, passions? Fed with the
> same food, hurt with the same weapons, subject to
> the same diseases, healed by the same means,
> warmed and cooled by the same winter and summer
> as a Christian is? If you prick us, do we not
> bleed? If you tickle us, do we not laugh? If you
> poison us, do we not die? And if you wrong us, shall
> we not revenge?

Fig. 7

question: should our baseline assumption in medicine be one of human sameness or difference? Humans have grappled with this question of centuries. Even Shakespeare engaged the debate, with Shylock's famous and manipulative argument for similarity between Jewish people and others in terms of anatomy, passions, and vulnerabilities. [Fig. 7] We need to keep asking the question now. I believe that our baseline assumption should be one of sameness, unless there is very good reason to think otherwise.

I am not a nihilist. Yes, of course there are some medically relevant differences between people of different ancestries. Tay Sachs disease is more common among people with Ashkenazi ancestry. Sickle cell trait is more common among people with West African ancestry. Buy as Jay Kaufman has shown, there is danger in applying these differences carelessly. Yes, sickle cell trait is 25-times more prominent in African Americans than in white Americans. But most African Americans don't have it. It would be wrong to treat all African Americans differently because of a trait that exists in a minority of them. And many white Americans have the trait as well. While 40,000 African American children are born each year with sickle trait, so are 6000 non-Hispanic white children. It is wise to consider the risk in all people.

Similarly, while it is possible to find genetic variations that correlate with race, something that provides reassurance to some that race is "real," this might reflect, in part, a sampling bias. Here's a thought experiment. If you divide a population into short and tall people, could you find genetic differences between them? I assume so. What about heavy or light people? Probably. What about Bostonians and San Franciscans? You would likely see differences in certain gene frequencies. Is race a more meaningful category than these others? That certainly depends on how you define meaningful. Should researchers

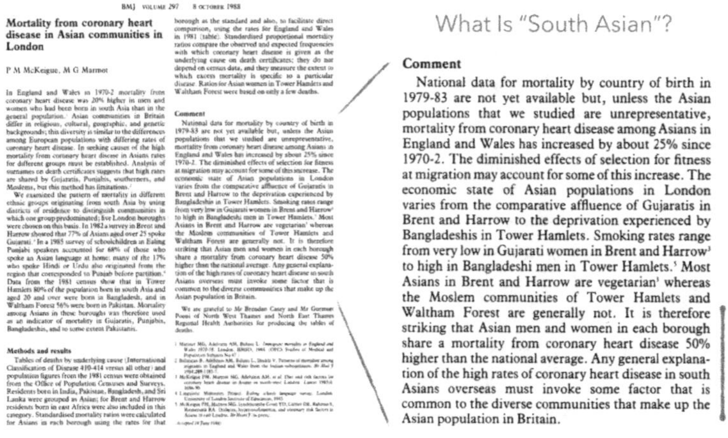
BMJ VOLUME 297 8 OCTOBER 1988

Mortality from coronary heart disease in Asian communities in London

P M McKeigue, M G Marmot

What Is "South Asian"?

Comment

National data for mortality by country of birth in 1979-83 are not yet available but, unless the Asian populations that we studied are unrepresentative, mortality from coronary heart disease among Asians in England and Wales has increased by about 25% since 1970-2. The diminished effects of selection for fitness at migration may account for some of this increase. The economic state of Asian populations in London varies from the comparative affluence of Gujaratis in Brent and Harrow to the deprivation experienced by Bangladeshis in Tower Hamlets. Smoking rates range from very low in Gujarati women in Brent and Harrow[3] to high in Bangladeshi men in Tower Hamlets.[5] Most Asians in Brent and Harrow are vegetarian[3] whereas the Moslem communities of Tower Hamlets and Waltham Forest are generally not. It is therefore striking that Asian men and women in each borough share a mortality from coronary heart disease 50% higher than the national average. Any general explanation of the high rates of coronary heart disease in south Asians overseas must invoke some factor that is common to the diverse communities that make up the Asian population in Britain.

Fig. 8

stratify populations by race, height, weight, and geography? I suspect we could often do fine without any of them.

In response to criticism, physicians increasingly acknowledge race as a social construct but then proceed to defend the continued use of race on new grounds. Race, they argue, actually useful as a proxy for racism. Race labels capture something meaningful about lived experience, about the ways in which exposure to racism is internalized and embodied, altering physiology. This is absolutely a relevant concern. But can you infer experiences of racism simply from someone's complexion or self-identity?

This raises the second part of the "what is race" problem: how we operationalize race. Here I think medical practice is deeply flawed. Many of the tools we reviewed relied on a dichotomous black-nonblack variable. Some upgraded this and used the US census categories of five races plus or minus Hispanic ancestry. This is neither scientific nor evidence based.

Consider three people, each of whom might arrive as Harvard freshman next fall. One might be a self-identified African American, descended from enslaved people, likely with 75% West African ancestry, who was born and raised Baltimore. Another might have been raised in an aristocratic family in Ghana. A third might be a second-generation Ethiopian immigrant born and raised in Boston. Do these three people have anything meaningful in common, either in terms of their ancestry or lived and internalized experiences of racism? Not necessarily. So why should our health care system treat all three of them as one type, distinct from other humans?

The same exercise could be done with South Asians. By the early 1970s, researchers had recognized high rates of heart disease in the South Asian diaspora, in Singapore, South Africa, or London. Sir Michael Marmot studied this problem and was flummoxed. As he explained, this increased risk made no sense. "South Asian" was not a coherent category, whether in terms of ancestral genetics, dietary exposures, or other cultural practices. [Fig. 8]

And the same exercise can be done with Hispanic. I am self-conscious, as a white guy from Boston, about telling an audience in California anything about the complexity of the Hispanic community. But I think we can all agree that there are people in the US who identify as Hispanic who have no shared continental ancestry (except in sense that we are all Africans). Cultural practices also vary across this category, depending on local background, degree of acculturation, and countless other factors.

The bottom line is that I have increasingly come to believe that the use of any of the common race and ethnic categories introduces a classic error of empirical research: garbage in, garbage out. Sine the categories and their implementation are flawed, I don't see how anything good can come from their use.

The fourth thing I want to emphasize is the harm done by these practices. Our ubiquitous, reflexive focus on race diverts attention from other factors that are relevant, arguably even more relevant than genetics. Consider pharmacogenomics, one of the first areas of genomic medicine that rose to prominence. The basic idea is sound: humans have many drug metabolizing enzymes and receptors, and these vary between people. Researchers jumped from that to a broader claim, that pharmacogenomic variants have a geographic, even racial distribution. As a result, we should prescribe differently to people of differ color. As Sally Satel wrote in the *New York Times*, "I am a racially profiling doctor." [Fig. 9, below]

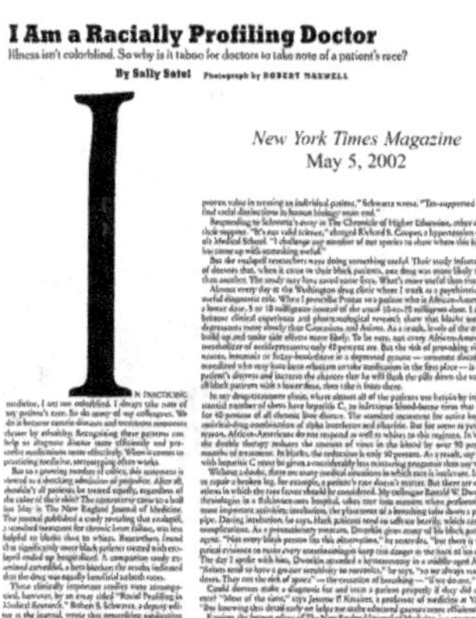
I Am a Racially Profiling Doctor
Illness isn't colorblind. So why is it taboo for doctors to take note of a patient's race?
By Sally Satel
New York Times Magazine
May 5, 2002

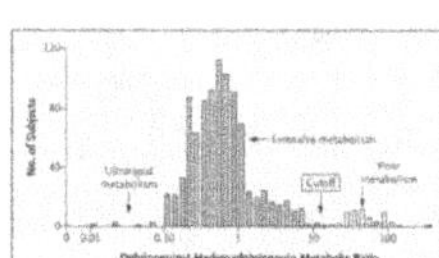

Figure 1. **Pharmacogenetics of CYP2D6.**
Urinary metabolic ratios of debrisoquin to its metabolite, 4-hydroxydebrisoquin, are shown for 1011 Swedish subjects. The Cutoff box indicates the cut-off point between subjects with poor metabolism as a result of decreased or absent CYP2D6 activity and subjects with extensive metabolism. Modified from Bertilsson et al.[17] with the permission of the publisher.

Weinshilboum, "Inheritance of Drug Response," *NEJM* 348 (2003): 529-537.

Table 1. **Pharmacogenetics of Phase I Drug Metabolism.***

Drug-Metabolizing Enzyme	Frequency of Variant Poor-Metabolism Phenotype	Representative Drugs Metabolized	Effect of Polymorphism
Cytochrome P-450 2D6 (CYP2D6)	6.8% in Sweden 1% in China[17]	Debrisoquin[15] Sparteine[16] Nortriptyline[27] Codeine[27,28]	Enhanced drug effect Enhanced drug effect Enhanced drug effect Decreased drug effect
Cytochrome P-450 2C9 (CYP2C9)	Approximately 3% in England[29] (those homozygous for the *2 and *3 alleles)	Warfarin[29,30] Phenytoin[31,32]	Enhanced drug effect[29-32]
Cytochrome P-450 2C19 (CYP2C19)	2.7% among white Americans[33] 3.3% in Sweden 14.6% in China[17] 18% in Japan[35]	Omeprazole[34,35]	Enhanced drug effect[36,37]
Dihydropyrimidine dehydrogenase	Approximately 1% of population is heterozygous[38]	Fluorouracil[39,40]	Enhanced drug effect[39,40]
Butyrylcholinesterase (pseudocholinesterase)	Approximately 1 in 3500 Europeans[41]	Succinylcholine[8,42]	Enhanced drug effect[8,42]

I think this is very bad medicine. Many of the alleles have small effect sizes. Most drugs are influenced by so many enzymes and receptors that the impact of any one variant might be small. The variants are typically found in just a subset of a particular group. Yes, one race or ethnic group might be at higher risk of being slow metabolizers of P450 2D6, but most members of that group have the wildtype allele. It would be wrong to treat all members of a group differently because of a trait actually held only by a subset of them.

Moreover, there are many things other than pharmacogenomic variants that have large effects on treatment outcomes. Cigarette smoking, for instance, upregulates many metabolizing enzymes and decreases the efficacy of drugs. One of my classmates in residency, Jennifer Derenne, now a professor at Stanford, cared for a woman with schizoaffective disorder. She helped her stabilize on clozapine, a valuable but dangerous drug that requires close monitoring of drug levels. During a period of relative wellness, she convinced the patient to quit smoking. Her drug metabolism slowed down, leading to a rise in her clozapine levels—and symptoms of drug toxicity.

Since the 1970s, researchers have documented many other ways in which life affects treatment outcomes. Diet, for instance, can have a large impact, whether leafy greens, grapefruit, or charcoaled meats. When we test drugs, we report outcomes by race and gender. Why not report them also by cigarette use? Meat consumption? Geography? Any of these could cause statistically significant differences in outcome.

Most dramatic of all is the impact of nonadherence. Estimates suggest that half of Americans are unable or unwilling to take prescriptions as instructed. You can prescribe according to race, or sequence your patients' genomes practice one mode of precision medicine. But you will likely have a far larger impact on your patients' treatment outcomes by having a serious and respectful conversation about their ability and willingness to follow treatment recommendations.

I certainly recognize that it is easier to criticize practices than to implement solutions. So I feel obligated before closing to make some specific recommendations. As I said earlier, I do not and have never called for color-blind medicine. As long as race and racism continue to structure access to wealth, health, and social resources, we need to study them. We should continue to include race in the descriptive statistics of health care. But we need to do a much better job with this. No good will come from dividing the world's people into black and nonblack. I don't know what set of labels is the best set, but researchers are working on that. Another option might be to drop such labels and rely instead on ancestry informative genetic markers. This too remains a work in progress, with a few intractable problems. But while I support the use of better race categories in descriptive statistics, I am wary of any use of race categories in predictive tools.

Meanwhile, any effort we invest in studying race, ancestry, and genetics should be matched, probably exceeded by, our attention to socioeconomic status. Too often studies say "we controlled for SES but a race signal persisted." How did researchers control for SES? Often by relying on a single, crude, static variable, for instance a 2- or 3-tier measure of educational attainment, or, less often, income quartiles. That is not adequate. Social epidemiologists have documented many relevant social exposures. We should document as many as possible. Moreover, it's not just the current measure that matters: what we really care about is the integral of SES exposures over a life time.

Yes, this will be difficult. But humans have accomplished many difficult things. The United States sent twelve men to the moon and brought them home safely. My colleagues at Harvard and MIT developed the country's two COVID vaccines in under one year. We have an incredibly resourceful and well-resourced scientific establishment. Surely we can solve this problem of descriptive statistics. We need to commit to collecting more comprehensive data about patients, both in research and clinical practice. We need to develop clever ways to analyze this data. But we can do this. Our patients deserve better than what we offer them now with race in medicine.

KIRSTEN BIBBINS-DOMINGO: Thank you very much. Dr. Jones, I'm happy that you provided two potential solutions in the end, but I want to push you a little bit more on one of the things that we do, at least at UCSF. As patients come in, we ask for their self-identified race and ethnicity. We ask other questions about their identity. We are trying to be conscious of how we use them in our clinical algorithms. What would be your recommendation to us for how we start? Do we capture more at the outset? Maybe the ancestry informative markers, maybe other aspects of SES, maybe the questions about racism? Or do we do more on the back end to make sure that we don't use it in the diagnostic and predictive algorithms? How should we be thinking given that we do have an urgency to address the health issues of our patients in the best way possible with the available information now?

DAVID JONES: I certainly agree that we have the urgency to do the best for our patients. The question is, are we doing that by foregrounding race or ethnicity as the sole or the key variable that we ask about in these things. When you look at medical studies that get published, in almost all of them stratify patients by age, by gender, and by race and ethnicity, and then stop there. That suggests that race and ethnicity are the key variable. I'm not going to deny that they have effects if you define them properly, which I don't think people often do. But there are many other things.

In healthcare, we never ask patients about income. Somehow, it's considered appropriate to ask patients detailed questions, intimate questions about sexual behavior, substance use, illegal activities. But somehow it's too uncomfortable to ask people about income. Well, why is that? What's wrong with medicine that somehow income is considered more intimate than details of your sexual practices? We deprive ourselves of important information about key variables that really do affect the lives of our patients. And now we just have this huge void in our knowledge set about how these socioeconomic variables affect things because we have not studied them as fastidiously as we have studied race, because a priori, we thought race was the key variable. And there are other political questions for why income-based measures have been excluded from traditional medical data sets. But this leaves us with really inadequate data.

We don't understand the things that really determine patient outcomes, or we choose to ignore the ones that do. As I said, noncompliance has an effect size that's much, much higher than almost any of the genetic effects that have been described so far. I mean, if we want to move towards precision medicine in the future, we need to enable a future that looks beyond genetics to other factors that alter outcomes. And doing these things would have a series of benefits that would de-center race from the role that now plays in medicine, decreasing the risk that medicine exacerbates activities. And I agree that this wouldn't be easy to do. We would need to rethink how we do research. But I really think our clinical research and our clinical practice needs to be motivated much more powerfully by structural competency, as Dorothy Roberts said, and not about assumptions of race differences as our guiding principle.

Moderated Discussion with Keynote Speakers

KIRSTEN BIBBINS-DOMINGO: So, these have been three fantastic keynotes. I want to say that we knew that there would be differences of opinion. Because Dr. Professor Roberts started us off, we are going to begin discussions by allowing Dr. Roberts to respond so that we can really have a discussion going and address the specific issues that Dr. Burchard raised.

DOROTHY ROBERTS: Right. Sure. So, I think that Dr. Jones did an excellent job of responding to some of the disagreements that Dr. Burchard had with my talk. So, I thought I would just mention a few specific points where Dr. Burchard explicitly said I was wrong or implied that I didn't know what I was talking about.

So, the first is that he said I was wrong in a statement I made about African ancestry, when I said that all human beings have African ancestry. And what is made up is where we count it as being part of someone, you know, determining someone's race. I never said anything about the migration out of Africa. I know that that has been estimated to be 20 to 50 thousand years ago. But what I was talking about is, at what point do we claim that human beings either don't have African ancestry or we don't need to take it into account? So Dr. Burchard's distinguishing between African Americans and Mexicans and white people, is in terms of African ancestry.

They all have African ancestry if we go all the way back far enough, to 50,000 years. So, at what point do we no longer have to count it in terms of determining their race? That's the question. And that is a made-up time period. That is, I have never found anyone who says exactly at what point after the migration that races were formed enough so that we can distinguish them, and we can distinguish African people from other people who do have African ancestry, but we don't have to refer to it. I hope that's clear. That is a completely made-up question.

It also raises the question, what distinguishes Mexicans and African Americans, if they have African ancestry? Right, if we go all the way back, what distinguishes them to be able to say, well, African Americans have African ancestry and Mexicans don't. Not only that, and not to get too personal, but how is Dr. Burchard's mother Mexican and not Black if she does have African ancestry? I could ask Dr. Burchard that as well. Obviously, that answer depends on a political or social definition of who is Mexican, who is Black. And we could say that about every single race. It's a made-up definition that there is no scientific or social consensus on, and that is one of the major problems with race-based medicine or race based clinical practice. Now, that's one point.

And another point – I'll try to go faster on the next one – is the idea that Black people are harmed if we don't take race, categorically and automatically, into account in either race correction or race norming. As Dr. Jones pointed out, they basically do the same thing. And there is evidence to show, as Dr. Jones points out in the article he referred to, but there are other articles as well, that Black people will be diagnosed later, not sooner, because of the race norming. They're denied claims as the NFL concussion settlement shows. Or they're denied being placed on a liver transplant waiting list because of race correction. So, it's not the case that if we take race out of these algorithms, Black people are going to be diagnosed later or misdiagnosed or denied treatment. There's evidence that it's just the opposite. And as Dr. Jones said, no one is saying to use a white norm as the norm for everybody. What we're saying is, figure out a better way of measuring these outcomes than relying on race.

And in fact, like in the eGFR, once we start saying we're no longer going to use these absolute categorical race distinctions, and the distinction between Black people and all other human beings, then that is when we start to find better ways of measuring these various functions. I also want to make the point, as Dr. Jones did at the beginning, that he is a trained physician, and he has studied this for a long time. As I pointed out, people might say that because I'm not a physician, I don't have anything to say on these matters. But I disagree with that. I would point out that the reason why race correction is getting left out of the eGFR in a number of hospitals now is because of the scientific, careful work of nephrologists who have pointed out that this is not good medicine, like Samantha Grubbs and like Amaka Eneanya at Penn.

KIRSTEN BIBBINS-DOMINGO: We're going to have a whole session on that.

DOROTHY ROBERTS: All right. It's just not true, though, that it's because of lack of training that people are arguing for ending race-based medicine. These are people who are well trained, and who have conducted excellent studies and know what they're talking about. Okay, I'll just say one last thing, because there was one other point where Dr. Burchard said I was wrong. I never said anything about epigenetics. I didn't use that word. So, I'm not sure why he said I was wrong about it.

ESTEBAN BURCHARD: I watched you talk in January 2021.

DOROTHY ROBERTS: A different talk. Okay, so let me just say that epigenetics, first of all, does not change genes at all. It changes the expression of genes, as I'm sure you know.

ESTEBAN BURCHARD: But it's inherited.

DOROTHY ROBERTS: There's absolutely no evidence it's inherited across multiple generations.

ESTEBAN BURCHARD: That's not true.

DOROTHY ROBERTS: Well, you're absolutely right that environmental factors that a pregnant person is experiencing, can cause epigenetic changes in the fetus. But there's no way we could know that epigenetic changes are inherited over multiple generations, because we have not studied that.

ESTEBAN BURCHARD: Yes we have.

[overlapping] DOROTHY ROBERTS: How could we possibly have studied if multiple generations haven't occurred since they started studying …

[overlapping] ESTEBAN BURCHARD We've studied it in mice. And it is an area …

[overlapping] DOROTHY ROBERTS: Oh, okay. Alright. Thank you.

ESTEBAN BURCHARD I mean, this is a topic that I'm familiar with. But let's talk about the first statement, about the one drop rule. It's self-identification. You know, I'm 5%. African, my mother is about 8%, African. But at the time, in the 50s and 60s, even though she was dark skinned, she was not considered African, she was not considered white. So the African American community didn't embrace her, even though she's darker than you. And the reality is, it's self-identification. And it's the Jim Crow law, which was implemented in 1800s and continued until the late 1930s, said one drop. So, if I had been born in the south, I would have been labeled African American, I would have been able to pass. And so, you know, there's a double standard within the white community and a double standard within the African American community.

DOROTHY ROBERTS: I absolutely agree with that. That's why it's not determined by ancestry.

[overlapping] ESTEBAN BURCHARD: I didn't say it was.

KIRSTEN BIBBINS-DOMINGO: Fantastic. One thing I'd love is to help us in our academic health centers here, and so I pose the same question I asked Dr. Jones. We have gone through a big effort at UCSF to ask people to self-identify their race. And we have talked about the problems with this. And one of the challenges in this entire set of discussions is when we should absolutely do away with this imperfect measure, or when we should understand its nuance and utility for some other things, perhaps even a marker of racism. How should we think about it, should we collect African ancestry or ancestry informative markers for all our patients? Should we do self-identified race, but just be careful on the back end on how we use it? Should we collect other measures? Dr. Burchard, and then Dr. Roberts.

ESTEBAN BURCHARD: Well, ancestry informative markers is a way-outdated technology from 2000. We can now use genome-wide estimates of ancestry where we use millions and millions of genetic markers. And each allele frequency difference, the cumulative allele frequency difference, mathematically can be used to cluster individuals.

KIRSTEN BIBBINS-DOMINGO: Is it something we should do on all patients when they come to the door?

ESTEBAN BURCHARD: Yes.

KIRSTEN BIBBINS-DOMINGO: Because it's important for discovery, or because it's important for how we care for our patients?

ESTEBAN BURCHARD: Well, what we clearly articulated in the *New England Journal* piece is that we don't know the answer. So, I'm a physician, well trained in epidemiology. And I know when to say I know and when to say I don't know. And so we said that it's an empiric question that needs further research.

KIRSTEN BIBBINS-DOMINGO Is it dangerous to measure all of these things – either Dr. Roberts or Dr. Jones – as patients are coming in the door?

Or, what should we measure as patients come in the door?

DOROTHY ROBERTS: Well, I think, Yes, as Dr. Jones said, there's no reason why we should identify people by race, as if it either has some innate information that helps to treat patients or that it's a proxy for some other important indicator. It would be much better to ask patients about what is important to their health. As Dr. Jones pointed out, whether they smoke, what their income is, what neighborhood they live in – those are more important than making assumptions about the patient based on their race. So, I would say we should think about what are the important factors that determine a patient's health, or might give a doctor some insight in diagnosing illness or prescribing medications and therapies and use those instead. Race?

KIRSTEN BIBBINS-DOMINGO: Dr. Jones, is it dangerous to do this? We understand that there's limitations to doing it. Is it dangerous to do self-identified race given that racism is a factor that influences health outcomes, and presumably, also influences those self-identified racial categories?

DAVID JONES: As I said, I have no problem collecting data on race and ethnicity in our descriptive statistics of medicine for the reasons you just said. We have to understand how these things are structuring outcomes. I think it is misleading and dangerous to collect that data and not collect all of the others, because that then creates an assumption that the only thing that matters to doctors is a patient's race or ethnicity. In American political discourse, as we've seen over the past five years or five centuries, many people operate as if they believe that there are fundamental differences between different types of humans. Why do they believe that? They believe that because scientists and physicians have been telling them that for centuries. We have to take responsibility for the impression that we have created in the public at large that there are fundamental differences between different types of humans, which is something that has a very pernicious effect on political discourse and human lives in this country.

ESTEBAN BURCHARD: Kirsten. I want to add that Jewish couples, for prenatal counseling, get genetically tested all the time. And it's because they're Jewish, because they have a higher inbreeding coefficient. And they're likely to have inborn errors, congenital errors, simply because their, quote unquote, racial or ethnic identification. So, it is something that we use all the time. And it's not a problem.

KIRSTEN BIBBINS-DOMINGO: Dr. Burchard, how would you respond to the concerns that are raised that, the limitations of other things and that other measures aside (and even the potential opportunity for discovery), that doing this continues to reinforce and elevate the ideas of biological views of race?

ESTEBAN BURCHARD: Again, I've reiterated it multiple times, it's an empirical question. As of today, we don't have a way to measure the biologic effects of socioeconomic status, cumulative lifetime experiences. I was born and raised in the Mission District, poor neighborhood, single mom, you know, the chance of me getting out was less than one in 10,000. I know the effects of poverty. I have scars on my forehead, on my eyes because of being beaten up in the hood. You know, of course, that's going to make me feel a little bit different. And also, it's going to get under my skin and causes epigenetic changes. But how do we integrate that experience, compared to someone whose parents are professors, in academics, and they start off life in a different stage of life than I did?

KIRSTEN BIBBINS-DOMINGO: Dr. Jones?

DAVID JONES: I would say, we don't know that, because we haven't made a serious effort to try to study that. As I said, we've gotten people to the moon and back. We made two novel vaccines in a year. We can do extraordinary things if we set our minds to doing it. We need to put our minds to it. It'll be a 50-year project to create lifespan integral data. If we don't start tomorrow, we're not going to have that data in 50 years. It's a hard task. We have to do it.

And the comment about genetic testing in people of Jewish ancestry or in Jewish populations, we have to be careful about the words we use. There's a fascinating pair of legal cases – and Professor Roberts, as a legal scholar here, might be able to bail me out on this – about two wrongful birth suits for couples who both went for genetic screening. The couple that was of Ashkenazi ancestry was not screened for Tay-Sachs. Child was born with Tay-Sachs. They sued and said that they should have been screened for Tay-Sachs because any genetic counselor should know that Tay-Sachs is a disease with higher prevalence and people of Ashkenazi ancestry. They won that case.

The other case was a French-Canadian couple. The judge decided that a reasonable genetic counselor shouldn't have suspected that Tay-Sachs was prevalent in the French-Canadian population, and therefore, was not found to have committed a crime, even though any reasonable genetic counselor in Boston or places that have significant population of French Canadians understand the Tay-Sachs actually is seen in that population. And that was the case where the usual race-based practice, testing people differently because they're Ashkenazi versus something else, led to the birth of a child with a terrible disease. We shouldn't do it.

KIRSTEN BIBBINS-DOMINGO: So let me ask… I knew this panel would be too short. Let me ask each of you to quickly say, if you could wave your magic wand and help us to think in our medical school, what we should be doing and teaching and practicing, what would the ideal world look like in five years for you? What would we be doing different? And how would we be doing this? Is it more measurements? Is it less measurements? Is it more? What are we doing differently? Who wants to start? Dr. Burchard?

ESTEBAN BURCHARD: Sure. If I was an advisor to God, I think the highest determinant of health is socioeconomic determinants. I think socioeconomic position, education, access to clean water, are the top priorities as physicians and public health advocates.

KIRSTEN BIBBINS-DOMINGO: Excellent. Okay. Dr. Roberts?

DOROTHY ROBERTS: Well, I'd say we would stop using race as if it were a biological category, when it is an invented political system of governing people in an unequal society. We would understand that race is an invented category, that because of structural racism and other inequities that Dr. Burchard just mentioned, we have a nation that is currently marked by gross health inequities and other kinds of other kinds of inequalities. And we would be recognizing that continuing to use race as if it were biological impedes progress. It impedes social change. It impedes better medical practice. It impedes better biomedical research. And therefore, we must abolish using it. It's the only way we will be able to make the changes that we need to make to have a more equal society.

KIRSTEN BIBBINS-DOMINGO: Excellent. Dr. Jones, you have the last word.

DAVID JONES: So, I would hope that five years from now on the baseline assumption of what we teach our medical students and other health professionals students is that, for the most part, we are members of a common species, that our shared humanity is much more profound than our shared differences. To the extent that differences do emerge, many of them are driven by the kinds of socioeconomic exposures that Professor Burchard mentioned in his final comments. I think we need to do much more work to characterize those and their effects. And this will be very difficult work. But I hope we are up to the challenge. Again, I'm not a nihilist. I'll certainly admit that there are differences in allele frequencies between people with different ancestral populations, some of these are going to be medically relevant. I think we need to remain attuned to the existence of those and practice accordingly, where they exist. But I suspect that in the long run, if we had proper datasets on socioeconomic status, we would realize that the genetic differences that exist are of relatively modest importance compared to the many, many other factors that affect our patient outcomes. And I hope that the health care professionals will direct their attention in their effort towards those most important determinants of health.

KIRSTEN BIBBINS-DOMINGO:
Well, with that, I want to thank each of you. Dr. Bouchard, Professor Roberts, Dr. Jones, this has really been a terrific conversation and so many of the comments in the chat and the questions really speaking to their appreciation of each of you and your commitment to this work and the scholarship. Thank you again for starting us off.

Moderated Discussion with Responder Panelists

KIRSTEN BIBBINS-DOMINGO: Okay, well, we're going to go right into the responder panel. And we're really fortunate to have Dr. Catherine Lucey, Executive Vice Dean in the UCSF School of Medicine. And I'm going to turn it over to her to launch this responder panel of colleagues from across the UCs.

CATHERINE LUCEY: Thank you, Dr. Bibbins-Domingo, and I want to express my thanks to all the plenary speakers. It was a fantastic, fantastic session with lots of thought-provoking comments. And I actually thought, probably more consensus in some of the areas then might be evident just on first look, and I'd love to hear from our panelists about that. We're going to be joined now with a distinguished group of panelists. I'll introduce them briefly, when I ask them to speak at the outset. And I'd encourage all of you to make sure that you look at their very impressive personal biographies online, because all of them have done important work in this area and that's why they were selected to be here. They also represent all of the University of California Schools of Medicine. And I think they can help us think through today, the practical applications of some of the controversies and commonalities that we just heard from our plenary speakers. So, what I'd like actually, to start off this panel is to just ask each of our panelists to weigh in on sort of initial reactions or take home messages or even sort of lingering questions they had from the panelists. And, each of you, I'd like to take no more than one or two minutes, because we want to sort of get into some more dialogue with this. I'm going to ask that we start with Dr. Happy Araneta, who is a Professor of Family Medicine at the University of California, San Diego. What struck you most about these presentations, or what questions do you still have lingering that you'd like us to discuss?

MARIA ROSARIO (HAPPY) ARANETA: Thank you, first of all, for inviting me and for organizing this panel with rich discussions. What struck me the most is that they're all correct. All their perspectives are correct and appropriate for different situations. I work on type two diabetes in non-overweight Asian Americans. And so, just the recognition that we have high prevalence of type two diabetes, despite the absence of general obesity, we were able to change the screening guidelines to screen Asian Americans at a lower

BMI cut-point. Otherwise 1/3 of Asians with type two diabetes with have remained undiagnosed. And so the utility of these, is it race correction, in this case applies to the population that I work with. It applies to COVID as well, where if you look aggregately at Asians, it seems like they don't experience the same rates of infection and mortality, but if you separate Filipinos, specifically Filipino nurses in California, the case fatality rate is 1.2%, but as high as 26%, among Filipinos. So I think my perspective adds to more complexity about dissecting racial categories further, especially in Asians where we share the same placement in the Asian continent, but there is little shared in phenotype or language or culture among Indians, Chinese and Indonesians.

CATHERINE LUCEY: Thank you, and thanks for your work in this very important area. Next, I'd like Dr. Alicia Fernandez, who is a Professor of Medicine at UCSF and Director of the UCSF Latinx Center of Excellence, to weigh in on her insights from the plenary speakers. Alicia?

ALICIA FERNANDEZ: Thank you. I think I like to make three points, particularly for our students. One is that, the reason today is so important is that this is the big lie. This is how we physicians, we scientists, have been instrumental in justifying the oppression of people and in racializing people. Black scholars have pointed out how the Irish and others were racialized in Europe in order to justify their bottom step. So, this is the big lie and we are the chief justifiers of that lie. We are the big priests of racism.

Number two is how any person who studies immigrant Latinos will agree completely with Dr. Roberts, in many ways. In the 2000 census, 42% of Latinos said they weren't (quote) "some other race." It didn't work. Same thing in the 2010 census: over a third. What does this mean? It means that these categories, obviously as social categories, obscure rather than elevate some of some of the things. And that, in fact, many people have spoken have studied among Latinos, how people will place them into racial categories in the United States that the subjects themselves, the participants themselves do not recognize. And because of that, I use ethnicity, the word ethnicity and not race in my own work, and I've had to change it. The journals have not accepted my use of the word ethnicity, which is a social construct, to refer to African Americans for others. And that I think that remains really important.

The third point is the need to elevate complexity. And in that I completely agree. We had some interesting discussions in preparation for this. Many people say, oh, it's all socioeconomic status. And anyone who studies Latino health knows how that's not true. The Latino paradox is precisely the fact that, for

Latino immigrants at low socioeconomic status, often have one of the highest life expectancies and often better outcomes. So, what then can we say to our students? We can say, you can do this. It is okay to hold complex thoughts. It is okay to understand the role of racism, to understand that sometimes this is a useful shortcut in medicine, and most often it is not. It is okay to elevate complexity. And yes, you can do this, I realize that people want easy answers. And that's not where we are.

CATHERINE LUCEY: Thank you, Dr. Fernandez. I'd like to now turn to Dr. Helena Hanson, who is Professor and Chair of Translational Social Science and Health Equity at the University of California, Los Angeles. Dr. Hansen?

HELENA HANSEN: Thank you. I mean, so many wise things have been said today. And so, I think that what I'm about to say will simply reinforce, maybe from another entry point. But I want to contextualize this conversation by thinking about where we are geographically, and what that has to do with the medicine that we practice. So, rather than beginning with the question that we were provided as panelists, or as discussants, beforehand of whether race based clinical guidelines are necessary, I want to examine why the US is uniquely obsessed with race based clinical guidelines.

We sit in the country that spends the most on healthcare per capita of any country in the world and gets the worst health outcomes of any industrialized nation. Other industrialized nations that perform better on health outcomes and spending, such as Canada, Western Europe, and Australia are multiracial, and they have potent racism that, by the way, is often strengthened by colorblind ideologies that won't acknowledge race and racism in the public record. But unlike us, they invest in social medicine, and they do not invest the same energy in debating race-based guidelines. We may not know if investing in genome wide studies for all patients, and practicing medicine based on them will make a difference for outcomes. But we do know that addressing social and structural drivers of health strongly improves patient outcomes.

In my decade and a half of research on the use of race in US pharmaceutical development and marketing, I posit that two factors together lead us to the horrifying results that we have in this country. Okay, they're uniquely horrifying results. One, we have the most brazenly for-profit healthcare system among industrialized nations. And two, our for-profit healthcare, pharma and biotech industries that make up the largest sector of the US economic system, depend on a rigid racial hierarchy that structures our national political culture and our biomedicine. So, this hierarchy is supported by the genetic determinist ideology that dominates US biomedicine. And it feeds the commercial sale of individually consumable technologies and services to individual patients deemed a genetic risk, rather than public investments in health promoting public infrastructures and social systems.

Genetic determinism also feeds into a political discourse in which some racialized groups are deemed biologically flawed and less deserving of expensive technologies, particularly if they have less private purchasing power. So, I just want to end with three points.

One, we have to name and push back against the racial capitalism that undergirds our economy. The racial algorithms that we debate are used to decide who gets insurance coverage for, and access to, different forms of expensive treatment granted. So this is problem. But even more pressing is the fact that our country's racist politics prevent us from investing in health promoting social benefits and public resources, from supporting universal health care and from standing up to the expeditious ethnic racial marketing of pharma and biotechnologies that simply take advantage of our hierarchy of white middle class consumers who can buy the most newly patented technologies, and publicly insured black and brown people who constitute a secondary market for products that are for chronic conditions that they disproportionately have, largely due to their living conditions. And for products that are, that are about to go off patent from the standpoint of the producers.

Two, we need bio-social research. So, as Dorothy Roberts and David Jones mentioned, biology responds to social environment. In fact, we are a species that has evolved to adapt to complex social systems, our biomedical sciences should reflect that fact. Rather than pouring billions of dollars into research that assumes genetic determinism, we must invest in new paradigms like epigenetics, neuroscience, neuroplasticity, and microbiome research that examine how social environments shape human biology. And this will require collaborations between biomedical researchers on one hand, and social scientists who have the conceptual frameworks and methods to help invent new approaches that are up to this task—new scientific approaches, bio-social ones.

And then lastly, social sciences need to be included as basic sciences of medicine. Rather than lamenting the low level of sophistication about race that we have among biomedical researchers and practitioners, medical schools must invest in robust education in the social science of health inequalities and race, which would provide a conceptual basis for types of practice, such as what I had colleagues call structural competency, that enable clinicians to address community, institutional, and policy level drivers of health inequalities. We must also build a foundation of social science and medicine, to incentivize collaborations between biomedical researchers and social scientists through grants and training. Thanks.

CATHERINE LUCEY: Thank you, Dr. Hansen. Dr. Aleksandar Rajkovic is next. Dr. Rajkovic is a Professor of Pathology and the Medical Director and Chief of the Center for Genetic and Genomic Medicine at UCSF. Dr. Rajkovic, your insights from the plenary speakers today?

ALEKSANDAR RAJKOVIC: Yeah, I think that this was a very educational session for me personally. As a clinical and research scientist, geneticist, the two recent events in our society have sparked really reexamination on diversity, equity and inclusion, and also has been an eye opener that has made me think about race, the use of race in clinical genetics. As we have seen from the esteemed speakers, this is a difficult and complicated topic. And I would say that that's true across UC system as a whole. I personally think the debate we witnessed is very healthy and necessary.

For geneticists, our two formal societies, American Society for Human Genetics and American College for Medical Genetics, have stated that race is a social construct. And these conclusions really have come from a lot of large population based genetic studies that have shown that individual differences are greater than intercontinental differences. And that diversity is really a part of a spectrum and not a matter of discrete clusters. And most of the current genetics literature is now much more sensitive to any placing in replacing race and ethnicity with ancestry and populations to capture human diversity. In clinical genetics, we know that lack of diversity can influence interpretation of genetic results by returning results that are of unclear significance. We also know that self-reported ethnicity is an imperfect indicator of genetic ancestry. Substantial and disproportionate risk of recessive disease is now detected when carrier screening is based on ethnicity leading to inequitable reproductive care. Clearly a pan population carrier screening that is inclusive of all populations, probably would be a better solution. And as part of this series, there will be a discussion about the use of polygenic risk scores and the shortcomings of these scores because of inadequate diversity.

So, health equity in genetics requires including more diverse populations across all of our studies. And this is really important towards the ultimate goals of personalized medicine, which is to optimize health at the individual level. Therapeutics that are genotype based are on the rise, and we need to understand the spectrum of genotypes across populations. And my recommendations to our students is really to question everything and apply appropriate methods to determine if current race-based measurements are actually needed or not.

CATHERINE LUCEY: Thank you, Dr. Rajkovic. And our final panelist for the initial reaction part of this panel, Dr. Ruth Shim, who is Professor of Clinical Psychiatry, and Associate Dean of Diverse and Inclusive Education at the University of California Davis. Dr. Shim?

RUTH SHIM: Thank you, Dr. Lucey, and I'm so pleased to be here with all of these experts. I'm going to keep my comments relatively brief, because I really want to engage with the attendees that are that are here today. I think that the reason that we need to reconsider race-based medicine is because of the application. Because our providers and faculty and our schools of medicine, we were all taught to believe that race-based differences are biological. So we were taught to believe in this concept of biological determinism. And that's because most of our physicians do not understand the nuances of race in the ways that we've been discussing them here today.

The UVA study on medical students that came out recently that Professor Roberts discussed related to this belief in biological determinism in the modern era, in the fact that in our medical schools now, students believe that there are biological differences between Black people and white people as it relates to nerve endings and skin thickness and pain. And so, it helps us to understand that knowledge in the hands of people who do not have expertise, and critical race theory, or race or racism, can be dangerous, due to implicit bias and structural racism. Because of structural racism, these beliefs lead to policies and practices that perpetuate and exacerbate health inequities, which Dr. Jones described. So Dr. Lea Davis of Vanderbilt described in a recent op ed in *Scientific American* that the field of genetics needs to have a reckoning with its past racist history. And I would argue that genetics needs to do this, but also the entire field of medicine needs to do it as well.

CATHERINE LUCEY: Thank you, Dr. Shim.

I'm the Education Dean for the School of Medicine, and what our students have challenged us to do on a daily basis is to get better. But I think it's misguided to lay the responsibility for this work at the feet of students. I think we are in a position where we must change the current practice of medicine to be more scientific, meaning to not consider races as deterministic and biologic. And I think we have to start changing the way that we as faculty, we as practicing physicians, we as leaders of institutions, look at race in medicine.

Race is unquestionably important in medicine, because it's important to patients, it's part of their lived experience. But that doesn't mean that we need to equate that with biologic importance. I think the conversation today sort of showed us how imprecise race is in characterizing individuals, and we run the risk of continuing to use statistical discrimination where we try and treat people as we treat populations, and that's not right.

So, I'd actually like the group to have a conversation about what do we do for the existing practicing physicians who have not actually heard this nuanced conversation today? How do we both educate them and create structures that protect vulnerable patients from misguided decisions based on people who don't have the sophistication around these controversies and challenges and race conscious medicine? I'd like to open up just for a general conversation what we do today for practicing physicians so that we become part of the solution and we don't just wait for a generation of students who have been educated appropriately to come into their professional practice.

ALEKSANDAR RAJKOVIC: So maybe I can say. My thought is, there's something that I have been very interested in and engaged with our societies about: why are we using race corrections for certain variables and for certain measurements? And what is the basis behind it? And should we actually be using it or not? And I think that we need to engage with societies that issue guidelines and are followed by students and clinicians. And so I think that this has to occur at the highest level in order to make significant change in the practice of medicine.

CATHERINE LUCEY: So you're sort of suggesting that we do away with race correction or race norming. Is that what you're suggesting, Dr. Rajkovic?

ALEKSANDAR RAJKOVIC: Well, I'm not going to say that we do away, but we should question, as has been suggested, and review what is the basis for these measurements. And this needs to be at the level of professional guideline committees, initiatives, guidelines that medical students and physicians follow. Those are where the changes need to occur, those levels, to make an impact.

CATHERINE LUCEY: Dr. Hansen?

HELENA HANSEN: Yeah, I'd like to respond to that. I think that would be very worthwhile. This comes back to a discussion that we have had amongst ourselves in preparing for today about whether to focus narrowly on race based guidelines for clinical treatment, or whether to broaden the scope. And I insist, we must broaden the scope because this kind of intervention won't make sense to practitioners unless they have a foundation in the social study of the creation of racial categories, and how racial categories that are called into question (and race based guidelines) are part of a larger institutional and ideological system.

And we've gotten a little bit of a glimpse of how we might move forward with that in the past year, because academic medical centers and leading clinical journals, including *New England Journal of Medicine*, have suddenly been using terms like structural racism, when they have not been in the past. And this is a direct result of organized political protest and pressure. I just want to say that right up front. Race is a political category, and it's taken political organizing to change the way that academic medical centers are approaching race. And they are amongst the more conservative institutions in our country. And I insist that it's because there's a lot of money at stake. There's a lot of political power at stake in biomedicine. And so, I insist that we cannot limit ourselves to a statement about the need to reexamine racial guidelines in diagnosis and care. We have to actually begin CME.

You know, you're talking about practicing physicians. If they haven't gotten it in medical school, or in their training otherwise, then CME credits need to be required so that they can benefit from the deep and long social scholarship based on very robust methods and conceptual frameworks about the social origins of race and racism in our medical system and in our country. So, I insist that that is a knowledge-base that biomedical practitioners must have. So, we have to have a conceptual foundation. And we have to have biomedical practitioners appreciating that there is a robust scholarship that, until now, has been explicitly excluded from medical education and practice. We have to bring that in and we have to draw on the current moment of political organizing and pressure to make sure that our academic medical centers require, and our certification bodies require, practitioners to be equipped, not only with what the racial guidelines are for diagnosis and treatment, but what is the conceptual framework.

You know, we spent time in medical school understanding the molecular basis for the medications we prescribe, and for the organ failure that we diagnose. We spend absolutely no time, I can certify you, in almost every academic medical center, except for perhaps historically Black medical schools, no time on structural racism, no time on the social scholarship that's incredibly deep and profound around this. So that's what we have to do. We have to have a foundation, we can't just surgically implant this kind of discussion about race based guidelines. It has to be on the basis of a knowledge base, to practice biomedicine that includes this scholarship.

CATHERINE LUCEY: Thank you. Other comments? Dr. Shim? And then Dr. Fernandez and then Dr. Araneta.

RUTH SHIM: Yeah, I just want to agree with Dr. Hansen and say that, especially when we talk about the political position, or the political issue, that is race, and racism, we're really talking about power. We're really talking about power structures and hierarchies. And very few places are as hierarchical and as power divided as the medical institution, the institution of medicine, or even academic medical centers.

And so, if we're really serious about moving in the right direction on these issues, it requires the people that have the power to be able to make real decisions about whether or not these are issues that should be debatable, whether biological determinism is a debatable thing, or whether it's accepted that this is bad science and bad medicine. And so, you know, in my institution at UC Davis, we're having discussions about mandatory training of all members of the entire health system around issues of anti-racism in medicine, because we feel that that's a value that everybody needs to understand. This is something that that we all have to kind of work on and commit to learning more about. But that gets to our faculty, which I think catches up to where our students already are. But that doesn't get to the person practicing out in the world, who was educated within the system, that we've identified is relatively flawed.

I think that, just as Dr. Hansen mentioned, that that's where CME comes in. And I think, you know, that's where we have to think about our American Medical Association. All of our guild organizations have to be responsible for addressing this. We've seen recent examples of how these organizations have gotten this wrong, including, you know, prominent deputy editors of *JAMA* questioning whether structural racism exists in medicine. So you know, we have a lot of work to do. But I feel confident that we can make a concerted movement in this effort. And I agree it's the responsibility of those in power to move into structure.

CATHERINE LUCEY: I think Dr. Fernandez was next Thanks, Dr. Shim.

ALICIA FERNANDEZ: I too, want to agree with Dr. Shim and Dr. Hansen, and bring up two or three concepts into the conversation just to make them more explicit. I'm a practicing physician at San Francisco General. I see patients from all over the world. It's one of the two most diverse hospitals in the United States. And I think that we can go badly off the rails here, if we think that this conversation needs to be around the concept of race, as opposed to the concept of healthcare disparities. We are, as I mentioned, the keepers of the big lie, and the people who propagate the big lie, that not only are there big, important biological differences, but that other races and specifically Blacks are inferior, that's been held and so on.

But we are also the keepers of the medical system. And I mentioned that I was a physician, because in my 20 years of practice, I have rarely had to contend with the use of GFR or the use of PFTs and have managed to take care of physicians competently. I look forward to being educated on that subject. And I am neutral on how that should happen and look forward to that education. On the other hand, I contend with healthcare disparities every day. And so my question for us at UCSF with an incredible leadership in Dr. Lucey, Dr. Bibbins-Domingo, Dr. Talmadge King, is, I am glad that the chief medical officer at UCSF health wants to know whether or not we should use GFR or PFT.

But I wonder about whether or not it is a real. I know it is not okay. I wonder if we can put that same passion and that same feeling to ourselves when we send out emails about COVID-19 vaccines through mechanisms that systematically disenfranchise our more vulnerable patients, when we do or do not provide language concordant care, when we do or do not provide language access. In other words, there are two things we own in medicine. We own the biological degradation of other people and the biological understanding. But the other thing we own is our medical practice. And we systematically disadvantage vulnerable people. And that is where we need to meet every time we talk about race in medicine in those first two years, we need to talk about healthcare disparities. I'm talking too long, but let me say to the students, look up two words. Look up Lysenkoism, and try to understand that concept in the context of the discussion about GFR, and so on. And then try to elevate the notion of social inclusion and social exclusion. And the reason for that is that social exclusion causes disease, whether that be gay people from all races, or whether that be social exclusion, on the basis of class, or on the basis of racism, or on others. Thank you.

CATHERINE LUCEY: Thank you. Dr. Araneta?

MARIA ROSARIO (HAPPY) ARANETA: Thank you. What I'd like to see enrich in the curriculum of all of our UC medical centers is inclusivity and representation, where Asian Americans and Pacific Islanders comprise one out of seven Californians, but there is limited content in our curriculum about Asian American and Pacific Islander health disparities. Pacific Islanders have the highest COVID infection rates in the United States, in California, and in 14 states. But that's not included in the national narrative. Filipinos and Asian Indians have the highest prevalence of both type two diabetes and gestational diabetes in California. But that's not included. It's often limited to a lunchtime discussion.

So training our learners, a third of whom are Asian Americans, to be aware of health disparities, but most importantly, dissecting the etiology of these disparities, is essential in a the state with the demographics that we have. Understanding that the reason why Filipinos and Asian Indians have such high rates of diabetes is that they accumulate so much visceral adipose tissue despite having 24-inch waistlines. But would that be recognized in a clinic visit? And what's the reason for that? Is it poverty? Is it the fetal origins of disease? Or is it colonialism as former British and American and Spanish colonies?

And what are the implications on trauma and intergenerational trauma with the domestic terrorism that our Asian American students are experiencing now? What are what are the consequences on outcomes? And it's not just now. It's Chinese Americans being blamed for the bubonic plague in San Francisco over a century ago, and the refusal of access to care in hospitals in San Francisco. So they created the Chinese hospital. I think that kind of inclusion, that representation and then dissecting the etiology, which includes genetic, biological, social, racism, as well as colonialism as cumulative factors.

CATHERINE LUCEY: Thank you. I think what's really interesting about this conversation, again, is the way (to borrow the terms from Alicia early on) that all of you are embracing the complexity of these issues and also bringing it back to a population of people who have historically been marginalized and pathologized. And I think this is one of the challenges. When we begin to teach people about healthcare disparities, some of the current narrative really, really is truncated at a pathologization of the race or the genetic ancestry: Blacks have more this, Asian Americans have more that, without (as Dr. Araneta said) following through and saying, Why is that? If it's not related to ancestry or genetics or biologic basis, what is happening here?

I want to push you all a little bit, because I will be the last person to say education is not part of the answer. Education is definitely part of the answer. Required education, I think, Helena, you're right. Continuing medical education requirements exist. And California in particular has been very specific about what unique areas, palliative medicine, substance use disorder, require added attention. And I think that's definitely part of the solution. But let's be honest about this. Like with all areas of medicine, some people will have great understanding following education, some people will not really understand the nuances and some people won't bother with the education.

So, I want to push you all again, to think in terms of systems and structures, about what we could do as leaders of health systems, or as leaders of professional organizations, to structure a better approach to provide care for diverse populations while we are educating those who are educable, while we get to a tipping point, because we are far from the tipping point of understanding of the complexities of this. I'm just going to put that out there. And if we simply rely on diffusion of information, we will be having this conversation a decade from now, and we might be a little bit better. And that's being optimistic, I think. What are the things that we can do? What are the levers that we can pull? Is this a metric issue around quality and safety by vulnerable populations? Let's hear a little bit more about the systems or structures that leverage points that we might exploit to accelerate our work in this area.

HELENA HANSEN: Can I hop in here, just because I totally agree with you pushing us beyond education and classroom learning. I've devoted the greater part of the last five to seven years working with colleagues to promote this idea of structural competency, which is just one term for a whole host of approaches that other people do under other labels. But the idea is that we have to move beyond knowledge base and recognition and reinvent our forms of medical practice in order to address health inequalities. And so how do we do that? I think that it has to start with local experiments and recognition and supporting of examples of people who have reinvented that practice.

And I actually say, I hold up UCSF as a place undertaking a lot of these experiments and different types of practice involving real collaborations with community organizers and a lot of consultation along the way with the people most affected by health problems, about what's important to them. A whole range of things can be used, including Cultural Arts and community histories, and employing community health workers and people who have the condition of concern as members of clinical care teams.

There lots of these kinds of experiments cropping up across the country. Without putting undue burden on our trainees, they're actually initiated by trainees, and many, many times on the medical school side who reached out to collaborators who are members of affected communities in non-healthcare sectors, like housing agencies, Criminal Justice, schools, and also policymakers.

And I think the reason why trainees are often very prominent in this is that the incoming generation has more of a grounding, on average, in structures as drivers of health, then the older generation does. They're simply ahead of us in that. But I'm just saying that it has to be, in some ways, an elevation of organically developing collaborations that are reinventing clinical practice. Systematic theorization, about how and why they work and then propagation of these models of care. They have to be translated, not simply adopted without any attention to local context. But this is a long-term proposition. And I'm encouraged that at every academic medical center that I've gone to recently, I'm finding groups of people – they may not be in the majority, but there are very vocal minority – that are saying we're not satisfied with the form of practice that we have.

And it's a self-preservative act as well, because we as clinical practitioners are dropping out of clinical practice at record rates. We're burning out. We're reporting that the reasons that we're dropping out are the structural barriers to improving health outcomes among our patients. It's totally dissatisfying to practice in the current system. And so for our own preservation, we have to be engaged in reinventing health care. And there are national organizations, professional organizations – APA, AMA, AAMC, ACGME – that can promote this, that can specifically incentivize the practice of a different kind of medicine and a rethinking of medicine. But it's going to have to happen organically with practitioners who see one, do one, teach one and actively engage with partners outside of medicine.

CATHERINE LUCEY: Thank you. Other thoughts? Dr. Araneta?

MARIA ROSARIO (HAPPY) ARANETA: I'd just like to repeat what Dr. Hansen mentioned, and I think we have to depart from opportunities of learning in a classroom setting and have rich lessons to learn from community partners.

RUTH SHIM: I want to build off of Dr. Hansen and Dr. Araneta. I think that the way that I've conceptualized how that relates to structural competence, is that underlying the social determinants of health, which are responsible for the health inequities that we see in our society, are our social norms, or our beliefs about populations of people, and our public policies, or the laws and policies that govern the decisions that we make in society. And those policies and those attitudes and beliefs work together to create an unfair and unjust distribution of opportunity in our society, which leads to these differences in health outcomes that we see, which creates the social determinants that create the health inequities that we see.

So, if we are serious, then, about trying to change that, education is not really going to get us to where we need to be. But that's only one tiny little piece. The work has to be about changing the policies. And sometimes the policy can lead to a change in beliefs about populations. So the intervention has to be done at the level of policies, and that could be institutional policy. So it could be whether you use eGFR or not. That could be an institutional level type of thing. Or it could be the way I believe it should be, needs to be more large-scale policies in communities: in local governments, and state governments, and in federal governments, because all of these policies have an impact on health outcomes. So the idea would be then that if we're really serious about making these changes, and making these interventions, that we then have to start influencing the policy decisions that get made at the federal, local and state levels. So as physicians and as providers, we need to form stronger and more serious relationships with our political system.

And, you know, I'm here in Davis. I'm located in Sacramento in the Capitol, and I don't have the reach or the connections that I should, given if I'm wanting to make these changes. We're not trained on any of this in medical school. But this is work that is critical to advancing the direction that we need to go if we're really serious about changing things.

CATHERINE LUCEY: Yeah, I agree. I think part of the role of education is to create citizens who advance our truly democratic values, not the tacit ones that sometimes we adhere to. Alicia?

ALICIA FERNANDEZ: I completely agree with Dr. Shim and my colleagues. And I want us to focus on getting our own house in order. We own healthcare disparities. We own health care disparities. We can change healthcare disparities. We can change healthcare disparities without changing the federal policies and laws. Not completely, because the internal logic of how you make money and how a health system keeps going is partly driven by that. But there is an enormous amount we can do.

I would like my residents and students to have a more complex understanding of race and ethnicity, yes. But I want people to say it is intolerable, intolerable that a hospitalized patient will be five days in the hospital, and no one will talk to them because they don't speak the language. I want people to say it is intolerable, that I get 15 minutes for a 20-year-old with a sore throat, and I get 15 minutes for my seven-year-old with diabetes, hypertension, COPD and CHF. And that I have very few mechanisms by which to impact that outcome. I want to say that we are actors in creating poor health.

And that while social determinants affect who gets sick and with what, once people are sick, we are the ones who affect whether they get better or not. And I think in that way, whenever we have a discussion about race and ethnicity and what that means, I want us to say "race, ethnicity, and healthcare disparities," "race, ethnicity and healthcare disparities." And the reason for that is that we own these things. These are ours. We could change a lot of these things in weeks. And yet, we don't. Why is that? Is it because we, too, understand that these people are less than beat on the basis of their race on the basis of their national origin? Why is that?

ALEKSANDAR RAJKOVIC: So, I just want to bring up what Esteban said in terms of rating the importance to healthcare, which is the socioeconomic status. And, of course, race, which we all agree has very little biological meaning, but is a proxy for structural issues that have affect our health. You know, it's hard for a busy clinician to grapple with all these issues regarding the socioeconomic status, and how the environment which these individuals live, how it impacts their health. They just don't have the tools to deal with that. And I think that also the care has to be more holistic.

You know, we have a lot of determinism. And although some things are in our genes, a lot of things are not in our genes. Actually, most of the stuff is not in our genes. And so we physicians cannot be alone in this. This is a societal issue. And I do think that also what we do as physicians is very much influenced by what is happening in the society. If pandemics and riots did not happen, we may not be having this conversation today. I think that there are a lot of things that have pushed us forward to discuss these issues that are very relevant.

And so, I think as physicians, we need to find partners, and we need to find big partners, influential partners, because by ourselves will not be able to solve this. Let us not kid ourselves. This goes way beyond the hospital and physicians and their practices. So again, I think that this is an important topic, but individuals, we can all of course try to make the change either with our societies or either criticizing guidelines or we're trying to change things which we think are actually racist in our environment. We can definitely do that. But the bigger changes will require large partnerships for this to happen.

HELENA HANSEN: I just to underscore what Dr. Rajkovic and Shim have raised – we absolutely have to pay attention to the top down as well, and our role in that. And Dr. Fernandez mentioned that as well. We own this. We are health experts. We are often quite absent when it comes to policy with a big "P" and advocacy, or on the wrong side of the fence. And this is a window of opening. We are definitely going to be talking about health reform for many, many, many years to come. But this this particular moment in history, we have a window of opportunity.

And we can definitely work with collaborators who understand policy advocacy, use our symbolic capital as physicians and other health practitioners, to advocate for reimbursements, for health care system that rewards population health outcomes, that rewards the narrowing of inequalities in health, that democratizes the control over health care, bringing in people from affected communities, people who are directly affected by health conditions into decision making at institutional levels. You know, we got a taste of that with performance-based reimbursement. But we can be at the table and really help to push this from the top down as well as from the bottom up. So, I just want to heartily agree with that. And we need policies and our participation.

CATHERINE LUCEY:
Thank you. You know, what's been fascinating to me is that this conversation very appropriately is looking at the spectrum of responses that we need to take to address the persistent and pervasive problem of both health and healthcare disparities in the United States. And in many ways, we sometimes get trapped into a very small area of controversy. And it's like the old story about, why are you looking for your wallet under the lamppost, if you lost a block away? It's because the light is better here. And so, thinking about interventions at the policy level, at the institutional policy level to Dr. Shim's point, also requires individual practitioners to understand that, fundamentally, a person's race is not their risk. There are many, many factors that we need to help people think about more holistically, and perhaps that's the approach we need to sort of start pushing at the individual clinician level as we're working on policy changes, global education, and redesign of medical education as well.

ESTEBAN BURCHARD: I firmly believe that being Black is a risk in our society for police differential effects. It is disgusting that 400 years later, we're still seeing it.

CATHERINE LUCEY: Yes, I agree with that. What I was referencing was a risk factor for disease. Skin color is not a risk factor for disease.

ESTEBAN BURCHARD: [The shooting of] Ahmaud Arbery is a disease.

CATHERINE LUCEY: Thanks. Agree. Dr. Dehlendorf?

CHRISTINE DEHLENDORF:
Yes, we have a question from the audience. How do you reconcile the problematic definitions we use to define race in clinical trials while also wanting to create diverse study populations and reassure communities that the interventions we study will work in different communities?

HELENA HANSEN: I bet my colleagues have a lot to say about this because they have so much experience working with communities that are affected. But the way to reassure communities in my experience is not necessarily to say, "oh, we're following x y guideline for your community." Because many of the communities that we're concerned about that have been very poorly served by us, they don't have a good experience with our practice or our guidelines. That's not reassuring. What's reassuring is the way that we engage with them and bring them to the table to discuss what's important to their health, and how we should be structuring our healthcare to address that. So, you know, I guess the question, which is a really good and provocative one, for me, it points to a misunderstanding of where trust between healthcare providers and communities comes from. I'm thinking of the largely black American and Latinx patients that I work with. It's not a matter of coming to them and saying, but I'm following the latest guidelines from my national professional organization. It is, what kind of relationship are we establishing, and what values with regard to following their lead and what's important to them when we convene.

CATHERINE LUCEY: I think maybe a follow up on that is look at the way we have normed populations because of studies that have been done in predominantly male, European, the descendants of European, ancestry that become the norms. I think the question is, how do we reestablish norms to broader populations? I think Dr. Rajkovic referenced that earlier. Is there a strategy, Aleksandar, that you think makes sense to allow us to begin to understand better what clinical trials should be looking at from a diversity perspective?

ALEKSANDAR RAJKOVIC: Well, I think, going back to Esteban's studies, I think that the binary slots of racial categorizations are totally imperfect and inadequate. I think that using ancestry will give us a much wider spectrum of the diversity of the populations, as Esteban was showing. Everybody's going to be different by ancestor. We're all individuals. We're different from each other significantly, and I said interindividual differences are, are larger between then between the Intercontinental differences. So, I think that race may be a proxy for socioeconomic and socio and structural racism experiences, which are also difficult to quantify. But I think our clinical trials have to involve diverse populations from the get-go. And I think NIH has started to actually require, for every grant or trial or enrollment, that you show that you have diverse populations that are either reflective of the community you live in, or are reflective of the United States as a whole. But I think we need to drill that deeper. And perhaps ancestry is one way of doing it. But you know, maybe others will have some suggestions and how, what that diversity should be defined as.

CATHERINE LUCEY: Thank you. Dr. Shim?

RUTH SHIM: Yeah, I just have two thoughts related to the question. And it really gets to this ongoing debate about how do we get communities of color to be more interactive with our research, and how do we do build more trust in the research that we're doing and making sure that there are more diverse populations in research. I think of it as two important concepts. One is cultural humility. Melanie Tervalon and Jann Murray-Garcia talk about how, if you're going to practice cultural humility, one, you have to look at hierarchies that are in place and be committed to dismantling hierarchies between the provider and the patient. And I think that we could look at those same hierarchies in the ways that we've conducted research traditionally, and asked if those models of hierarchies are correct, which I don't believe that they are. I think they need to be dismantled.

But then the other tenant of cultural humility is this idea of partnering with communities, truly partnering with communities – not go and grab someone from the community and put them in a powerless situation, where they have absolutely no influence on or informing of the work. So that is not the type of research or partnership that is most effective. I see the solution as a workforce issue. So innately again, medicine is hierarchical. It has been exclusive. And the people that have been able to make it in medicine, save for a few people of color, are majority dominant population folks majority, and in leadership positions, majority men.

I think that the work that needs to be done is to get more physicians of traditionally excluded, of oppressed and minoritized backgrounds into the fields of research, because they don't have these same issues. They don't have these problems. If they're coming into the work to work in their communities and help their communities, there is an innate desire to partner equally. So the work that needs to be done, it has to be on the workforce level, but for the existing providers, the existing researchers, they need to be thinking more from a cultural culturally humble perspective.

MARIA ROSARIO (HAPPY) ARANETA: There also has to be an acknowledgment about the inherent biases involved in participating in and intentional recruitment in clinical trials. So often, I'm a local PI of a 26 site, multi-center study, where in the final analyses, Native Americans, Native Hawaiians and Pacific Islanders, and Asian Americans – their data are dismissed because the sample sizes were too small. And the response in our communities is, well then why were we enrolled in the first place? And the perception is we are the providers of healthcare, but there's no interest in our disparities. The Asian American Pacific Islander population is 6% of the national census. However, only 0.17% of NIH dollars are invested in health disparities research among our communities.

CATHERINE LUCEY: Thanks. Dr. Burchard?

ESTEBAN BURCHARD: I can't show my video. But, I want to echo Dr. Shim's point. We need more minority physicians and more minority scientists. Currently, African Americans make up 4% of the physician workforce. Latinos make up 4% of the Latino workforce. In California Latinos make up 50% of the state populace. And just, that number has not changed in 40 years. I started medical school 32 years ago, and that number has not changed. And we need to make a big dent in that, because as Dr. Shim had pointed out, those individuals tend to gravitate – and it's been shown over and over and over – they tend to gravitate to see minority patients and do research in minority communities.

CATHERINE LUCEY: And I think to add to that, Dr. Burchard, it is critically important that our faculties become more diverse, that we don't just strive to diversify the entire physician population or health professional population, but the people who are going to be driving research, educating the next generation, leading healthcare systems through the transformation needed, have to have people who have been in minoritized populations at the table with those decisions. We are almost out of time. Maybe one wrap-up comment from each panelist and then am I turning it back over to Kirsten?

ALICIA FERNANDEZ: To our students, I would say this – elevate intellectual complexity, elevate complexity in all of its forms, and position yourself with a true north. Complexity doesn't mean that there isn't a true north. It's not about our words, it's about our actions, and specifically, place ourselves at the service of our disenfranchised, of our vulnerable patients.

CATHERINE LUCEY: Thank you, Dr. Hansen?

HELENA HANSEN: This is probably another way of saying what Dr. Fernandez just said. We need a scholarly base so that we can really understand those complexities of race and who has been left out of the paradigm that necessarily has been anti-Black racism in this discussion. There is a whole history. There is a whole ideological underpinning and political underpinning to the medicine that we practice. And one thing that's distinctive about physicians of color, is that they tend to be curious about that. They tend to, because of their lived experience, reach for that kind of scholarship. It should be a basic foundation for medical training and practice. And so, I just want to elevate the complexity, and that we need the scholarship to inform that complexity because right now we're operating with very simplistic conceptual foundations in biomedicine.

CATHERINE LUCEY: Thank you, Dr. Rajkovic?

ALEKSANDAR RAJKOVIC: Yeah, I would like to say that disparity doesn't lie in our genes. Disparities are societal, socioeconomic, and I think that, in order for us to make everybody benefit, we need to encourage diverse populations, and their participation. That unfortunately, comes with obstacles because some populations are very worried about scientific research and how it's used. And I think that engaging communities, diversifying our workforce, diversifying the scientific workforce as well as physician workforce, as has been discussed, is so important to increase that engagement and that participation.

CATHERINE LUCEY: Thank you. Dr. Araneta?

MARIA ROSARIO (HAPPY) ARANETA: Twelve months ago, it felt like the world was awakened when COVID disparities amplified the structural inequalities that affected communities of color. But sadly, twelve months later, we're still seeing these inequities in vaccine allocation. Awareness doesn't always translate into equitable outcomes. To the students, I say, remain your strongest advocates, partner with allies from disciplines that you rarely interact with, because that's how we learn. That's how we partner. Create your own advocacy labs, learn from the ethnic studies departments, from the political science, from lawyers, from the community organizers. But don't be complacent.

CATHERINE LUCEY: Thank you, Dr. Shim, the final comment from panelists. Thank you.

RUTH SHIM: I actually just want to elevate Dr. Jones's words, that he said before, that this is hard work. This is a big task that we are setting out upon. But we have done hard things before. And so, I've said this before, that I remain skeptically optimistic about our ability to make change and move forward in this area.

CATHERINE LUCEY: I know from the many, many questions and comments, on the Q&A, how very valuable our audience has felt this conversation has been. And people are here from all levels of the medical profession and other professions as well. So I think that the work you've done today, and the presentations you've made, and the discussions you've led, really are going to move us forward in a very deliberate way and prepare us for the next set of seminars in this series. So with that, I'm going to turn it back to Dr. Bibbins-Domingo, who was the brainchild and the innovator around this series, and let her have the final comments for today.

KIRSTEN BIBBINS-DOMINGO: Great, that was really phenomenal panel discussion. I appreciated the morning, and then also appreciated my colleagues here from across the UCs broadening us to the discussion. I think that there are many questions and seeing our audience so engaged this entire time, I think speaks to the importance of this topic.

I loved the call from Dr. Jones and then from the rest of you to embrace the nuance, that we're up to the challenge and can actually do the hard work that needs to be done. To train the next generation to provide the best care for our patients, and to conduct research that will ultimately provide knowledge for everyone. I want us to, as we close out and look forward to the next sessions, to think about how we take the broad concepts that we've had today and really think about the decisions that we are all faced with on a day to day basis; to think about the decision that we made to take the race out of the eGFR; and the subsequent conversations we had to have about how reasonable it is for us to make more COVID testing available to Latino patients, because we know that there's a disparity there.

What does that mean to have those conversations? How can we be fluent as a community in understanding what one decision is and the implications for other decisions? What does it mean when we say race is a social construct, but we want to diversify our clinical trials? Why do we want to diversify our clinical trials? What does that mean for us to say that that is a goal that we as an institution have to do? What's the basis behind that? And I think that these aren't questions that have easy or right or wrong answers, but they are the ones that I think we struggle with every day to communicate with our colleagues and amongst ourselves. And as Dr. Lucey said, to communicate, not just with those of us who thought a lot about these issues, but with all of us as we try to create a community of scholars and practitioners.

So, we have many more sessions to continue these discussions. My hope is that you will continue to have these discussions in your own groups and on your own end. The next two sessions are asking us to grapple with the specifics that go behind the decisions that we make every day in medicine. Our case studies on April 7 will look at race, racial categorization and racism in medicine today, starting with a clinical vignette, and then several really outstanding speakers. We are going to continue with case studies on the 14th including on eGFR and on polygenic risk scores and ancestry. And so I would urge you to join those discussions. Session four, another Wednesday still to be determined, we're going to drill down deeper into the specific mission areas that are important to all of our campuses.

Thank you very much.

Introductory Remarks

Kirsten Bibbins-Domingo, PhD, MD

KIRSTEN BIBBINS-DOMINGO: Good morning. Welcome to our series, Racism and Race: The Use of Race in Medicine and Implications for Health Equity. This is the second session in our series, sponsored by the UCSF School of Medicine in partnership with our sister schools of medicine across the University of California. My name is Kirsten Bibbins-Domingo. I am the Vice Dean for Population Health and Health Equity in the UCSF School of Medicine. I'm delighted that you are joining us today.

Before we get started on this session, I want to comment on our first session, which took place two weeks ago, and really kicked off this series. We had three terrific keynote speakers and two panels that really kicked off our series and made up the bulk of the half day two weeks ago. We received a large number of comments about our first session, comments that appreciated the high quality of the outstanding talks and scholarship presented, appreciation for the broad expertise of the speakers and discussants and the exchange of ideas on both panels, and appreciative of the format and the venue for creating a conversation on the exchange of sometimes divergent views that we don't oftentimes get to hear in the same time and place. We also received concerns, including from those who appreciated the content, but the tone of the session was not always respectful. We agree. And these are comments that we take seriously. And so, I want to underscore two really important points.

The topic that we're addressing today, on the use of race and medicine, is a complex and nuanced topic that we are trying to unpack. We have intentionally brought together experts and scholars of this topic who have important perspectives that sometimes differ. Discussion, debate and disagreement are part of the scientific method, and we are appreciative of the willingness of these experts to engage in that work to advance our understanding of this important and complex topic. I am personally very fortunate to have learned from these presenters, many of whom are colleagues and friends who hold different views. Because many of us have learned and grown throughout this process of exchanging ideas, this is precisely the reason why we think these types of sessions are important.

Respect for our speakers and discussants is not only expected, but it is essential if we are to do this work. Our presenters are putting themselves out there on this important topic. They bring their scholarship and expertise. They also bring their own identities and lived experiences. It is critical that we listen to each other in a spirit of mutual respect, and do so in a way that more consciously sheds the multiple hierarchies of privilege that we bring to these discussions. These are hierarchies by race and ethnicity, by gender, by academic rank, by institution, and by discipline. Anything that prevents us from fully listening to each other on this important topic will also prevent us from doing this work effectively. So, these are the values that we are bringing to this work. Here's our shared values. The differences of opinion are expected and are welcome. All speakers and discussants are treated with respect. And despite different views, we have two common goals: advancing anti-racism in medicine, and pursuing health and health equity for our patients.

In this series, we are examining a small but important slice of race and racism in medicine – that is, how we use the concept of race in how we teach in how we practice and how we conduct research. We spent our first session laying the foundation with historical and current perspectives. And what we want to do in this session today and in our session next week is to examine a series of case studies to help us to apply principles and concepts that we've learned about to specific scenarios that we oftentimes encounter in medicine. This brings us to our fourth session on April 28, where we will try to stimulate a series of discussions within our mission areas, allowing for small groups to discuss the implications of our sessions for how we teach, how we practice, and how we conduct research. I want to highlight the fourth session, because we are really fortunate to have leaders from across our UC campuses, who've come together to think about the work we're doing today and what it means for how we think about race in medicine, from an education perspective, from our clinical practice perspective, and from the types of research that we conduct.

For our session today, we will follow a similar format to our last session. But we are focused today on a clinical case study. So we'll hear first a clinical case followed by a series of flash talks. There will be a panel discussion among the presenters, and then have a second panel discussion that will begin with a commentary and end with a closing commentary. I'm really grateful to Dr. Christine Dehlendorf, who is Professor of Family and Community Medicine, who has been a partner in co-organizing this event, and really is the architect for this particular session today.

The URL [at the front of the book] will take you to our website where a recording of today's session will be posted. You can see a recording of our first session, there's information about upcoming sessions, and there's today's agenda. We don't have time to do long speaker bios because we want to get to the content of their work, so I'd encourage you to read more about our speakers. And they have all offered a library of resources. So, there's an impressive library there as well.

Again, just the details of our upcoming sessions. On next week, we will continue with our case studies on eGFR glomerular filtration rate and on polygenic risk scores. Those are the two cases we're studying next week. And then again, session four on April 28, really going deep with our small group work in each of our domain areas. And so with that, we're going to move to the case presentation and flash talks.

Clinical Case Study

KIRSTEN BIBBINS-DOMINGO: I am really thrilled to have three outstanding colleagues of mine at UCSF who have agreed to give these talks that will follow the case presentation. Dr. Valy Fontil is an Assistant Professor in the Department of Medicine in the Division of General Internal Medicine at San Francisco General Hospital. He is a hypertension researcher and a faculty member in the Center for Vulnerable Populations at UCSF.

Dr. Michelle Albert is Professor of Medicine and Professor of Cardiology. She directs the Center for the Study of Adversity and Cardiovascular Disease, the NURTURE Center. She is the Associate Dean of Admissions in the UCSF School of Medicine. She is also the incoming president of the American Heart Association.

Dr. Akinyemi Oni-Orisan is an Assistant Professor of Clinical Pharmacy and Bioengineering and Therapeutic sciences in the UCSF School of Pharmacy. He is a faculty member in the Institute for Human Genetics, and a pharmacogeneticist. And we're really pleased to have all three of these outstanding presenters give their perspectives on the case study, and we're going to begin with a video of the case. [https://tinyurl.com/zp9xwjfr for Video.]

VIDEO NARRATOR: In recent years, medical institutions across the country have started to acknowledge that medicine has a race problem. Study after study has shown that historically marginalized racial groups shoulder a disproportionate burden of disease, have worse health outcomes, and experience substandard treatment from the medical establishment. So, what is race? How does it impact health? And how does it inform our clinical management of patients? And how does our understanding of race impact health equity?

As was discussed in the first session in the series, race is a social category, not a biological category. However, the fact that race is a social invention does not negate the reality that living in a racialized society has biological consequences for minoritized racial groups. We know for example, there is a higher prevalence of hypertension and diabetes, and a higher mortality rate from heart disease in Black Americans compared to white Americans. Since we have established that race is a poor proxy for genetics. These types of disparities are best explained by systemic racism, and the resulting lived experiences of those categorized as belonging to a racial minority group.

Environmental racism, discriminatory hiring practices, police violence, redlining, food insecurity, inadequate housing, to name a few, all disproportionately affect Black and brown communities, and can have profound impacts on health. So, given all this, how is race currently used in medicine? And how should race be used in medicine going forward? Let's examine some of the ways that race currently impacts clinical care with a hypothetical patient encounter.

Mr. Thomas is a 55-year-old man who presents to clinic to establish care. He has a history of hypertension and asthma and is not currently taking any medications aside from a rescue inhaler. His provider, Dr. Jones, talks to Mr. Thomas about his hypertension and together they decided to start medication therapy. Dr. Jones consults the JNC 8 guidelines for the best pharmacologic treatment options and shows Mr. Thomas the treatment algorithm.

DOCTOR [in video]: As you can see, your best option would be a thiazide diuretic or calcium channel blocker.

NARRATOR: While Mr. Thomas thinks to himself, Why does my race influenced my treatment options? My mother is white and my father is Black. Does that change anything? What other aspects of my care are affected by my identity? I've had bad experiences with healthcare systems in the past, and I don't want to seem combative or ignorant. So I won't ask any questions. He says, "Okay." Mr. Thomas is started on a fireside and returns to clinic A few weeks later.

DOCTOR [in video]: I'm glad to see that your blood pressure is better. today. I'd like to talk some more about cardiovascular disease. Given your age, sex, race, cholesterol and blood pressure, you have about a 13% risk of atherosclerotic cardiovascular disease, also called ASCVD in the next 10 years.

As you can see, Mr. Thomas, being Black significantly increases your risk of cardiovascular disease. In fact, putting in your race as Black gives you double the risk than if you were white.

MR. THOMAS [in video]: Why is that, doctor?

DOCTOR [in video]: Well, there are likely many contributing factors, but it probably boils down to genetics. Regardless, your risk is high enough that I'd like to start you on a statin.

NARRATOR: While Mr. Thomas thinks to himself, being Black intrinsically makes me less healthy? Is my body fundamentally inferior? He says, "Okay."

DOCTOR [in video]: Lastly, I'd like to discuss how well your asthma is being controlled with your current medications. Interestingly, some research shows that African Americans may respond differently to commonly use medications like inhaled corticosteroids and long-acting beta agonists. So this may require us to make some dosage adjustments to your medications.

MR. THOMAS [in video]: You know, I had no idea my race had such a large impact on my health and treatment options. Luckily, my asthma has been really well controlled with my current medication. So, I think I'd like to stick with that.

NARRATOR: As we saw with Mr. Thomas, race is commonly and too often uncritically utilized in various aspects of medicine. And a patient's race can directly impact the diagnosis, treatment options, and overall quality of care a patient receives. As clinicians and scientists, we must constantly question when, how and why race is employed. Some questions to consider are, in what circumstances is it appropriate to utilize race in clinical medicine? Should it be used at all? How might the use of race in various clinical scenarios perpetuate or alleviate inequity? And, how can we use race in a way that reflects an understanding that patients' experiences existing in a racialized society, not inherent racial susceptibilities, are what put them at risk for poor health outcomes? In considering these questions, we can understand how to use race in a way that is thoughtful, intentional, and critical with the goals of better understanding and addressing the root causes of health disparities, and ultimately improving the care our patients receive.

[End video presentation]

KIRSTEN BIBBINS-DOMINGO: Great, thank you. I'm going to invite Dr. Fontil to begin at the talks.

Hypertension

Valy Fontil, MD, MAS, MPH, UCSF

VALY FONTIL: Thank you, Kirsten. Again, my name is Valy Fontil, and I do research on hypertension. I'm really honored to be here and be part of this important conversation.

What I'd like to do first is to just clarify what we saw in the video as the guideline recommendations for hypertension with respect to race. Essentially, in the video, you saw that the guideline really said that, for a Black person or African American, that you should start therapy with either a thiazide diuretic or a calcium channel blocker. And what the guidelines in effect are saying is really to avoid an ACE inhibitor or angiotensin receptor blocker as the initial therapy for blood pressure treatment specifically in Black patients.

Is this race-based consideration for treatment of hypertension in these guidelines really warranted? And in thinking about this, I wanted to approach this and share with you simply just my thought process. What won't be included in this talk is a thorough review of the guidelines, or in-depth critical review of the evidence, but I hope by sharing with you the rationale, they can start to trigger a conversation and questions that will help us bring light to this topic. So are these guidelines really warranted is the question. And in answering this, I asked myself essentially five questions that I think is important to answering any of these types of questions. And the first one is what is the rationale and intention behind these? What's the underlying evidence? What's the quality of the underlying evidence? Are these specific race-based recommendations helpful? Is there a better alternative? And what is the potential harm of having this guideline? [Fig. 1]

So, the rationale that underlies these recommendations from some sort of epidemiologic studies [is] that Blacks have a higher prevalence of hypertension and lower rates of blood pressure control, and that there's evidence in the literature to suggest that Black patients tend to have a lower response to ACE inhibitors and angiotensin receptor blockers. So based on this evidence, many guidelines, at least more than six guidelines dating back at least to 2010, have suggested that ACE inhibitors and ARBs should not be routinely initiated as

Rationale

- Blacks have higher prevalence of hypertension and lower rates of BP control
- Evidence suggesting lower response to ACE inhibitors and Angiotensin Receptor Blockers

- Conclusion: ACE inhibitors and or ARBS should not routinely be initiated as monotherapy
  - OK to use them in combination with other drugs

Fig. 1

a model therapy.

I would also point out that it's really talking about initiating as a model therapy, but all the guidelines always point out that it's okay to use them in combination with other drugs, regardless of race. So, what's the state of the underlying evidence behind this? [Fig. 2] One is that what we mentioned before is ACE inhibitor monotherapy is associated with higher blood pressure in Blacks. The biggest criticism of the evidence is that there isn't sort of preset RCTs that had a direct comparison to study this question. But there has been multiple post-op analysis, pre specified post-op analyses, cohort studies, and some comparative effectiveness studies in real world practice, to suggest that this association is true, that in fact, Black patients on model therapy with ACE inhibitor tend to have higher blood pressures, when compared to whites. There's been a meta-analysis that shows this about a 4.6 millimeters of mercury difference. And a recent systematic review has also confirmed this racial difference in blood pressure response on model therapy ACE inhibitors

Underlying evidence

- **ACE inhibitor monotherapy associated with higher BP in Blacks**
  - No RCT direct comparisons, but
  - Multiple posthoc analyses and cohort studies
  - Meta-analysis (13 trials) – 4.6 mm Hg > Whites
  - Recent systematic review

- **Low-renin hypertension suggested as underlying mechanism**
  - Low renin = more resistance to ACE inhibitors and ARBs

Fig. 2

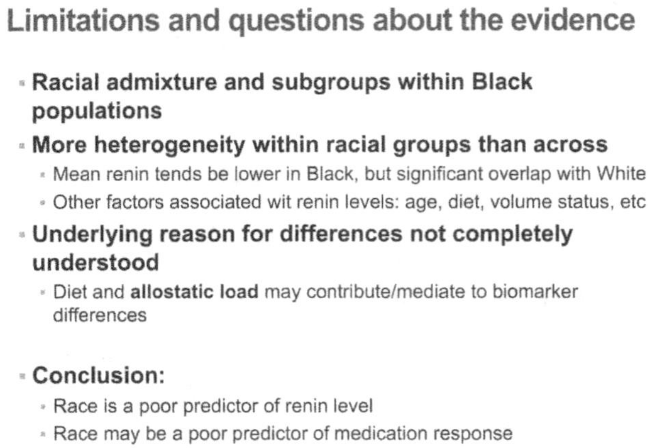

Fig. 3

or angiotensin receptor blockers.

The other rationale behind this is that lowering in hypertension is the underlying mechanism for this difference that we see and medication response. The idea being, low-renin state is associated with more resistant ACE inhibitors and angiotensin receptor blockers. I'd be happy to answer questions on this mechanism. But there's been multiple studies that have looked at the average renin by race and have shown that Blacks tend to have a lower renin levels, and that could explain this difference we see an ACE inhibitor efficacy in different races.

So what are the limitations and questions about the evidence? [Fig. 3]For one, there is this question of racial admixture in different subgroups within Black populations. I think that's a significant limitation because, as the person asked in the video, the question is, what about people mixed race? Do we see these associations in terms of blood pressure response? And the literature, in my view, does not really elucidate this. And then there's also the question of subgroups within the Black populations, in many ways, even geographic variation may not really fit this overall difference that we see. There's more nuance there that's understudied in the literature.

The second limitation is that, as I think we've discussed before, there's more heterogeneity within racial groups than across racial groups. And that's true for both response to blood pressure medications and in terms of the underlying mechanism of having low renin. So for example, the mean renin levels tend to be lower in Black patients, but there's significant overlap when you look at the distribution of renin in the Black population compared to the white population. The other thing that the recommendations miss is that there are other factors associated with low renin levels, including age, including salt

Significant overlap in response to Quinapril

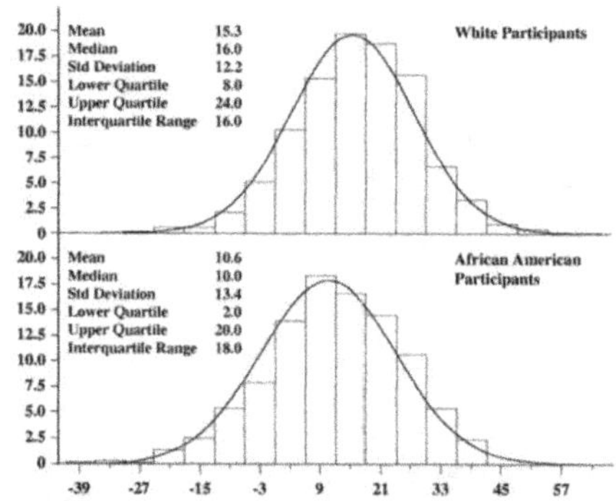

Evan Mokwe. Hypertension. Determinants of Blood Pressure Response to Quinapril in Black and White Hypertensive Patients, Volume: 43, Issue: 6, Pages: 1202-1207, DOI: (10.1161/01.HYP.0000127924.67353.86)

Fig. 4

content and diets, including volume status and other interactions. That makes you wonder why race was singled out as opposed to some of these other factors that are associated with lower response to ACE inhibitor therapy.

The next thing is, the underlying reasons for the differences are not completely understood? We know that there are interactions between genes and environment [that] contribute and contribute to these differences. The other thing is the concept of allostatic load just in terms of just experienced racism, experienced psychological stress affects the physiology in a way that would, that could confound or at least contribute to this relationship.

So in conclusion, I would say that race is most likely indeed a poor predictor of renin level if you think about it, and is likely also a poor predictor of medication response with respect to ACE inhibitors and angiotensin receptor blockers. Just to illustrate this point, in one study that was looking at Quinapril that compared the response to Quinapril, which is an ACE inhibitor, between whites participants and African American participants, you can see here that you see the difference. [Fig. 4] So the median response in Blacks is 10 millimeters of mercury, and the median response for whites is 16. And so you see this difference in the response. But if you look at the actual graph, one, you see that the distribution is wide in both groups. In each group is very wide distribution in whites and very wide distribution in African Americans. And significant overlap, if you were to juxtapose or these two curves together.

And so just to drive this point further, what this says is that there are a lot of white patients and white participants who don't respond that well to ACE inhibitors. And there are a lot of Black participants who did get good response to ACE inhibitors. And so there's a significant overlap there, that kind of gets

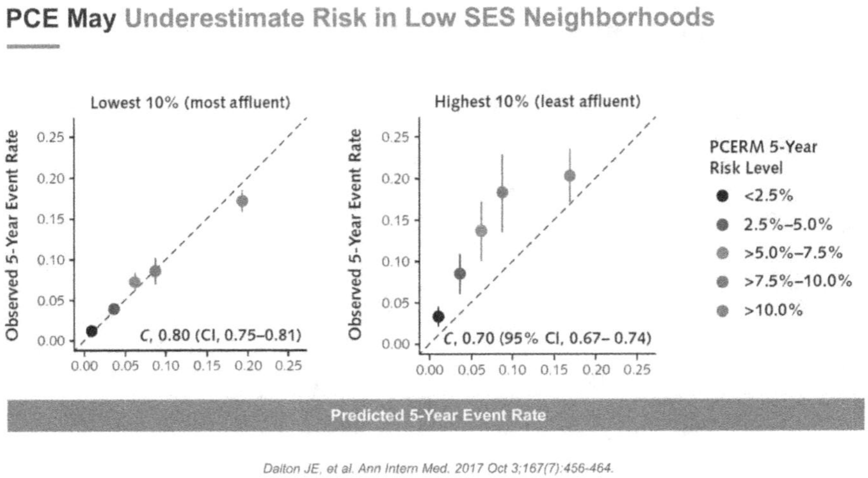

Fig. 5

lost in the recommendation and interpretation of these.

So the next question is, are these recommendations helpful? Is it helpful in reducing disparities? I've not seen much evidence that it is. [Fig. 5] You know, these regulations have been around. There's some evidence that doctors are actually following these guidelines. And we don't see a trend in reduction in disparities as a result of this. And I'm not surprised by this, because if you wanted to reduce disparities, focusing on which medication to use is probably the wrong focus. In clinical practice, it's not super helpful because it's really difficult to implement in practice. How does a doctor actually determine a patient's race? How does that doctor communicate that treatment plan to the patients? What is the potential harm? [Fig. 6]

Well, one potential harm that I like to highlight is that this could lead to suboptimal therapy, frankly, in non-Black patients as much as with the Black patients. So, one of the most immediate potential harm is that it could lead to inappropriate use of ACE inhibitor monotherapy in non-Black patients. There's also a risk that you can inappropriately avoid ACE inhibitor in Black patients who actually need it. For example, patients with certain kidney disease, specifically proteinuria.

You know, a doctor may make the mistake in thinking, well, we can't use ACE inhibitor in Blacks and therefore avoid that. It would be a mistake, but these guidelines make it more likely that that physician would make that mistake. It may reinforce a cognitive bias based on skin color, and potentially detracts from more appropriate priorities, like rapid escalation of treatments. Most patients in general, and Black patients in particular, will require two

Potential harm

- **Suboptimal therapy Black and non-Black patients**
    - Inappropriate use of ACE inhibitor monotherapy on non-blacks
    - Inappropriate avoidance ACE inhibitor therapy in blacks who need it
- **My reinforce cognitive bias based on skin color**
- **Potentially detracts from more appropriate priorities**
    - Rapid escalation of treatment – 2+ medications
    - Policy interventions
        - Food access
        - Transportation
        - Mental health services

Fig. 6

or more medications. And so the focus and the biggest barrier is sort of the timidity to be to escalate treatment in these patients. And also, it detracts from the real important priority of policy interventions that addresses social determinants such as food access, transportation, and also mental health services.

I would also point out that there is a better alternative to focusing on this. [Fig. 7] I think the evidence would lead us to focus more on ACE inhibitors and ARBs and not really race. The truth of the matter is that ACE inhibitor monotherapy is just probably a poor choice for many patients. And that we should consider avoiding ACE inhibitor monotherapy in most patients who don't have kidney disease or heart disease, and we should think about ACE inhibitors and ARBs generally best as used in combination with other things. So, you know, in the end, I would say that these guidelines are not warranted, and that guidelines to avoid monotherapy ACE inhibitor and ARBs in Black patients are, frankly, unnecessary, and potentially misguided or harmful.

A better alternative

- Focus on ACE inhibitors and ARBs, not Race
    - ACE inhibitor and ARB monotherapy may be a poor choice for a plurality of patients, regardless of race
    - Consider avoiding ACE inhibitor monotherapy in most patients without kidney or heart disease
    - ACE inhibitors and ARBs generally best used in combination with other drugs

Fig. 7

KIRSTEN BIBBINS-DOMINGO: Thank you very much, Dr. Fontil. I'm going to turn it over to Dr. Albert to comment on the case study using race in our 10-year predicted probability of cardiovascular event.

ASCVD

Michelle Albert, MD, MPH, UCSF

MICHELLE ALBERT: Thank you. Hello, everyone. The goal of my presentation today is to contextualize the 13% CVD 10-year risk in our patient, and also to hopefully provide a lens into the future for risk assessment for cardiovascular disease and stroke.

I wanted to start with the principles of ASCVD risk assessment. It is important to realize that risk assessment offers the doorway, and is not an end all be all, and focuses on absolute risk that is prognosis versus relative risk, which is dependent on our reference incident rate of a condition in the population. It seeks to identify persons at higher risk of getting atherosclerotic disease and those who might receive enhanced benefit from therapies such as statin therapy, aspirin therapy and blood pressure control. And also focusing on where the number needed to treat to achieve a particular risk reduction is low. It starts clinician patient discussion, such as how intensive preventive therapy should be.

I also think that it's really important as we think of the CVD risk score to think of the history of it. [Fig. 1] On this slide, you can see that there are nine risk scores that were put forward in the United States starting in 1998 to our present time, starting with the Framingham score. It is important to realize that the Framingham included persons of European descent [who were] white men and women and no individuals of color or no Black persons. So in the development of the pool cohort equation ASCVD risk score, the focus was to make sure that it represented a population of whites and Blacks and this convened a work group in the NHLBI and included four multi-ethnic cohorts, including the Atherosclerosis Risk in Communities, the Cardiovascular Health Study, CARDIA, and the Framingham Health Study.

So that is how our pooled cohort equation was derived from a population perspective, and then there's a contemporary cohort validation utilizing the REGARDS cohort. I was honored to be one of the writing group members of the most recent 2019 ACC/AHA guidelines for primary prevention of cardiovascular disease, which recommended use of the pool cohort equations

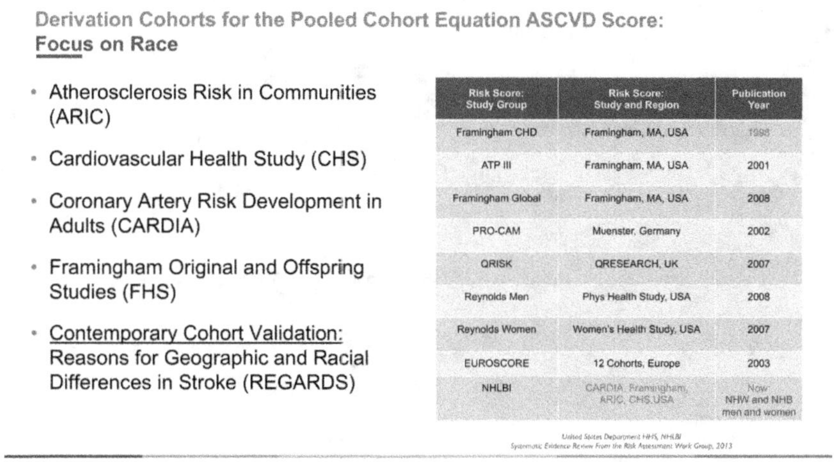

Fig. 1

as the first level of assessing cardiovascular risk.

As we think about cardiovascular risk assessment, the PCE is validated in non-Hispanic whites and non-Hispanic Black persons living in United States. [Fig. 2] The guidelines also now have clear language about limitations of the PCE – the PCE may overestimate or underestimate risk. As you can see in bold on the right side of the slide, the things here – age through hypertension – are included in the risk score. However, other very important factors that impact risk are not. And you see on the right-hand side of the slide, including therapies, including pregnancy related CVD, socioeconomic factors, mental stress, depression, etc.

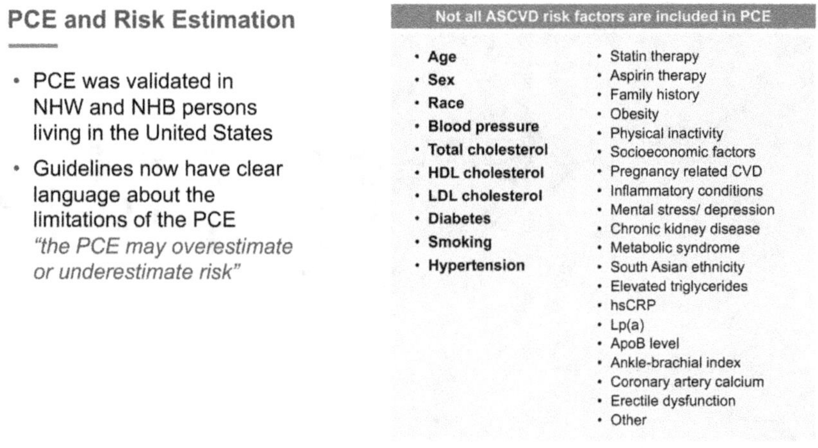

Fig. 2

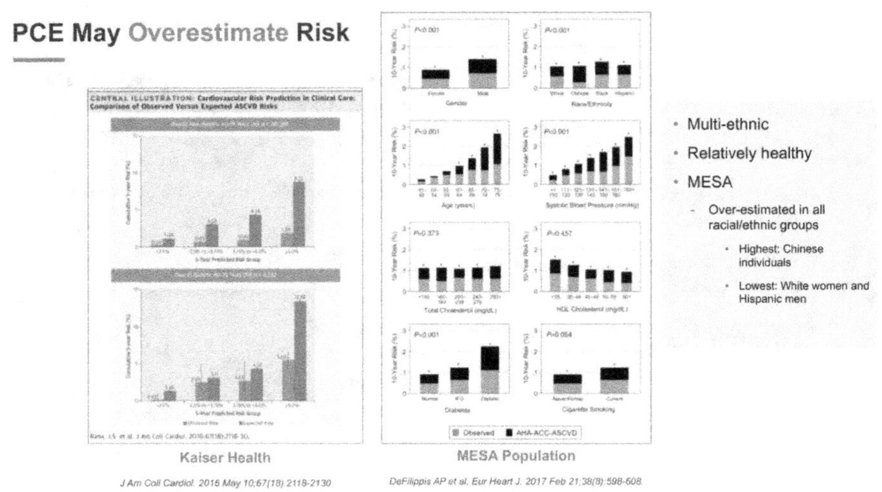

Fig. 3

So where might the PCE overestimate risk? [Fig. 3] We know that the PCE overestimates risk in relatively healthy individuals. So these are data from the Kaiser Health, showing in red that the expected rate of CVD is much higher than the observed rate in a relatively healthy cohort – that is, folks who did not have diabetes, did not have high cholesterol levels, etc. And then in the MESA study, the PCE over-estimated risk in all racial and ethnic groups. The highest over-estimate was in Chinese individuals and lowest in white women and Hispanic men. PCE also underestimates risk in those persons with inflammatory conditions. So just HIV, rheumatoid arthritis. [Fig. 4, below]

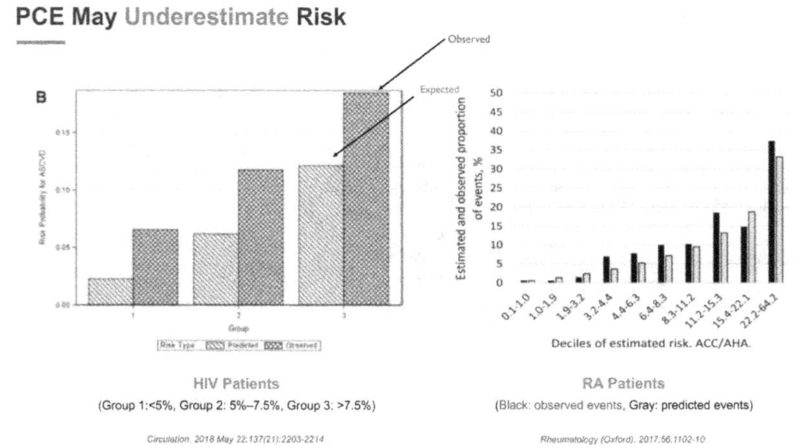

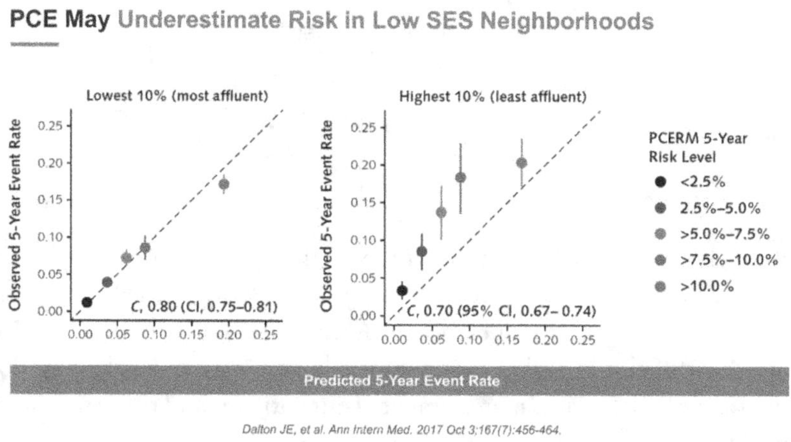

Fig. 5

If we take into account social determinants of health, such as neighborhood SES, PCE also underestimates risk. [Fig. 5] On the right-hand side of the slide, the dotted line shows the predicted risk. And in the least affluent neighborhoods in this study, published in the *Annals of Internal Medicine* 2017, you can see that at every risk level, the observed risk of persons living in the lowest neighborhood SES was much higher than what the PCE predicted versus those in the most affluent neighborhoods, the risk prediction was spot on the expected line, the observed risk.

In the 2019, ACC/AHA guidelines, there are several general recommendations for care. [Fig. 6, below] Team-based care, shared decision making, and for the first time, the guidelines included that social determinants of health should be used to inform optimal implementation of treatment recommendations. I should note that it didn't say anything about social determinants of health incorporated in predicting risk. Social determinants of health are important in risk assessment, and this was recognized by the guideline writing committee because we know that socioeconomic disadvantages are

Recommendations for Patient-Centered Approaches to Comprehensive ASCVD Prevention
Referenced studies that support recommendations are summarized in Online Data Supplements 1 and 2.

COR	LOE	Recommendations
I	A	1. A team-based care approach is recommended for the control of risk factors associated with ASCVD (S2.1-1–S2.1-14).
I	B-R	2. Shared decision-making should guide discussions about the best strategies to reduce ASCVD risk (S2.1-15–S2.1-18).
I	B-NR	3. Social determinants of health should inform optimal implementation of treatment recommendations for the prevention of ASCVD (S2.1-19–S2.1-25).

$$\text{CVD Outcome + Well Being} = \frac{\text{Adversity + Resilience}}{\text{Wealth}}$$

Albert MA
https://nurturecenter.ucsf.edu

Fig. 7

not captured by CVD risk equations. Indeed, there was a recommendation that the Medicare/Medicaid-developed screening tool – [used] to assess social determinants of health including housing instability, food insecurity, transportation difficulties, utility assistance needs, and interpersonal safety – be considered as we look towards management of our patients, and risk assessment. There were example considerations for addressing social determinants to help prevent ASCVD. And so for example, in cardiovascular risk assessment, the recommendation was made to evaluate psychosocial stressors, pay attention to health literacy, as one attempts to implement management and therapies for patient, pay attention to economic factors, neighborhood environment when one thinks about exercise on physical activity, for example.

It is really critical to understand that social determinants are linked to adversity. The definition of adversity from the Merriam-Webster dictionary is that it is a state of serious or persistent difficulty, a calamity or misfortune, that affects one's ability to achieve various goals, outcomes and well-being and happiness. Certainly in our case for Mr. Thomas, there was no discussion with Dr. Jones about underlying factors that might impact his preventive care.

This is an equation that I came up with, to think about how does adversity translate into clinical medicine. [Fig. 7] If we think about outcomes in this case: CVD outcome plus wellbeing is the balance of adversity plus resilience

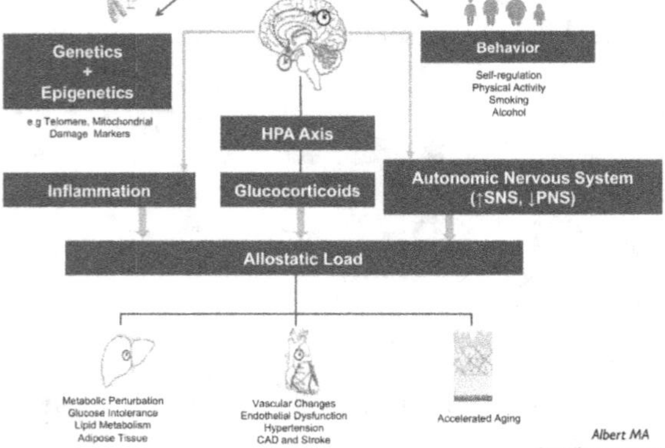

Albert MA
https://nurturecenter.ucsf.edu

Fig. 8

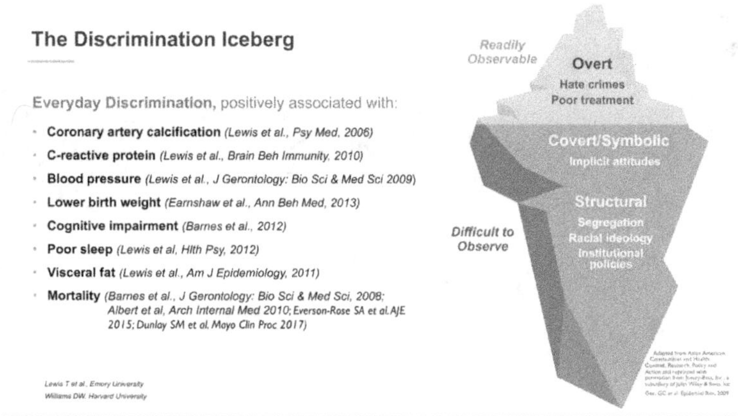

Fig. 9

over wealth. And wealth can be joy, it can be money, it can be however one defines it. As we think about this issue of race and racism, I would like to argue that the biology of racism related adversity gets baked into our brain, resulting in various biological processes, upregulation of inflammation, glucocorticoids, our fight or flight response, resulting in biological short circuiting, or allostatic load resulting in cardiovascular disease, metabolic perturbations, such as diabetes and accelerated aging, all influenced by behavior, as well as genetics and epigenetics. [Fig. 8]

Certainly, we know from the cardiovascular perspective that the discrimination iceberg is really important. [Fig. 9] We know that discrimination can be covert or symbolic, which is about two thirds of our discrimination. And you'll hear some stuff about structural discrimination, which is key, as we think about, you know, risk prediction and healthcare. And there's readily observable or overt discrimination. We know that everyday discrimination is possibly associated with surrogate biomarkers of cardiovascular disease risk, including coronary artery calcification, high levels of C reactive protein, hypertension, as well as one study showing mortality, visceral fat, poor sleep, and cognitive impairment. So getting back to our patient, what factors should influence our preventive strategies? Can we trust the PCE? Or do we need to do more? Certainly, Mr. Thomas has agreed to take a statin. But it can be argued he should be reluctant to take the medication based on what we know with regards to a medical mistrust for therapies, as well as the use of race in medicine.

Certainly, from a practical perspective, what we have right now is assessment through PCE, thinking of 30-year, ASCVD risk, adding risk enhancing factors such as metabolic syndrome, chronic kidney disease, and

Our Patient:
ASCVD Risk Calculation – Race Comparison

	Black		White	
	Male	Female	Male	Female
10 Year	13%	7%	6%	3%
Lifetime	50%	40%	50%	40%
Optimal	5%	2%	4%	1.4%

- Middle of the range of Intermediate Risk: Lifestyle, BP Control, Statin
- Risk Enhanced: ? Inflammation (Asthma)
- Meet Patients Where They Are: " What are their preferences/priorities?"

Fig. 10

adding coronary calcium to our risk assessment toolkit in order to determine what therapies and advice should we give Mr. Thomas. So as it pertains to the risk assessment, and the race comparison, you already heard that for Mr. Thomas, his 10-year risk is twice that of a white male. But I want to remind us about intersectionalities that exists as well. [Fig. 10]

If Thomas was a woman, a Black woman, her 10-year risk would be 7%. That is also based on a PCE, two times higher than a white female. However, as you heard, this biology of adversity, or racism related adversity is what probably determines this risk. And the question we have to ask ourselves if we were to add the social determinants of health into our risk equation instead of race, is how would it affect these numbers? Nonetheless, what we're left with, for therapy for Mr. T, is that his risk assessment falls in the middle range of risk.

So we would recommend lifestyle, blood pressure control and statin. And we need to ask yourself, is this risk enhanced from inflammation? He does have asthma, which is an inflammatory condition. And you'll hear more about that in the next flash talk. And it's important to meet patients where they are. That is, understanding what their preferences and priorities are. So to conclude, I would say that ASCVD risk assessment is a bridge over troubled waters. The points here are that the guidelines are evolving related to the ASCVD guidelines. And the recognition that social determinants of health especially underscored by racism categorizes persons in a manner that has real biological consequences. And that equity depends on understanding and capturing social risk in assessment and management. Thank you so much for inviting me to be a part of this discussion.

KIRSTEN BIBBINS-DOMINGO: Thank you, Dr. Albert. I'm going to turn it over now to Dr. Oni-Orisan and to talk us through some of the aspects of this case related to pharmacogenetics.

Pharmacogenetics

Akinyemi Oni-Orisan, PharmD, PhD, UCSF

AKINYEMI ONI-ORISAN: All right, my name is Akinyemi Oni-Orisan and I'll be talking about pharmacogenetics, race, ethnicity, and genetic ancestry. So, as you saw in the case, the patient was told by their clinician that they'd respond differently to asthma medications based on their race. The patient was also eligible for statin therapy based on their race, and actually, I will be focusing on that treatment, as opposed to asthma medications. The question here is, how can we optimize standard therapy to maximize benefit and minimize risk?

We first turn to the 2018 ACC/AHA cholesterol guidelines. [Fig. 1] So the guidelines recommend moderate or high intensity standard therapy, depending on the clinical factors of baseline ASCVD risk, and this really pertains to efficacy of the therapy. However, stands also cause side effects, most commonly muscle toxicity. And so this warrants further optimization of the therapy. This is where pharmacogenetics comes in. The previous guidelines, the 2018 ACC/AHA guidelines really didn't have any pharmacogenetic experts on the reading group, so that wasn't really addressed. However, the clinical pharmacogenomics implementation consortium, based on substantial

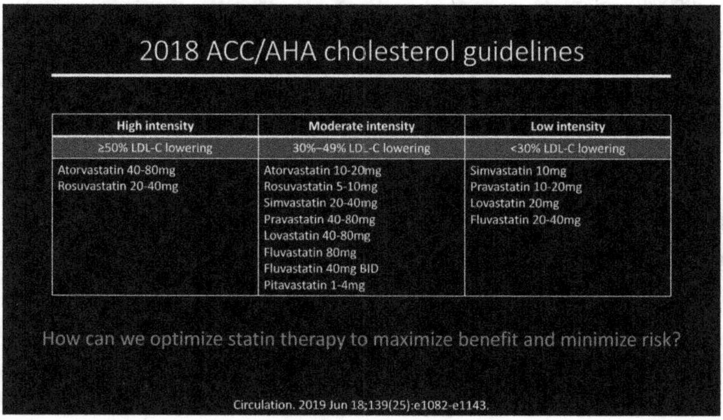

Fig. 1

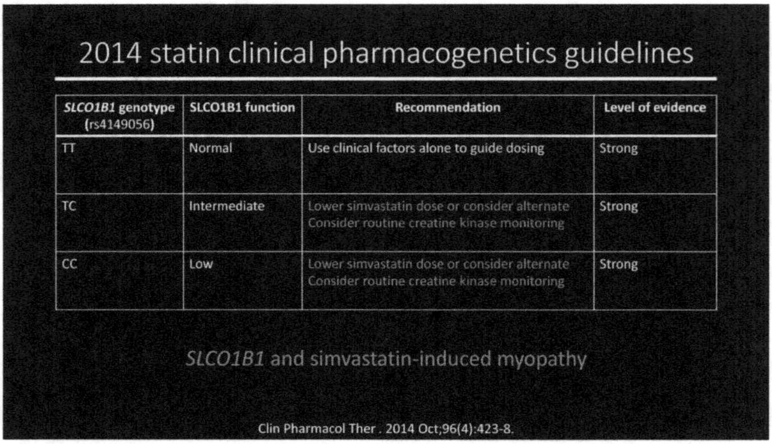

SLCO1B1 genotype (rs4149056)	SLCO1B1 function	Recommendation	Level of evidence
TT	Normal	Use clinical factors alone to guide dosing	Strong
TC	Intermediate	Lower simvastatin dose or consider alternate Consider routine creatine kinase monitoring	Strong
CC	Low	Lower simvastatin dose or consider alternate Consider routine creatine kinase monitoring	Strong

Fig. 2

evidence, has recommendations on how we should guide statin prescribing based on genetic background. And they recommend, with a strong level of evidence, that individuals with intermediate or low function in a gene called SLCO1B1 should be prescribed lower simvastatin dose, or consider alternate statin therapy due to increased risk of statin-induced myopathy, a 16-fold increased risk in individuals with this CC genotype, a really large effect size. [Fig. 2]

Pharmacogenetics is the effects of genetic variants on how someone responds to a drug, whether that be efficacy, safety, or how the body processes the drug. And so how exactly does this occur? The genetic variant can impact how the drug is absorbed, how the drug is distributed throughout the body, how the drug is metabolized, how the drug is excreted, pharmacokinetics. And the genetic variants can affect how the drug binds to a receptor at its target site, pharmacodynamics. So one of the most important concepts in pharmacogenetics that we try to teach is that this is only one piece of the puzzle. There are many other factors which impact how someone responds to a drug.

In addition to genetic variation, adherence plays a role, kidney function or other organ function, concomitant medications, even the microbiome, even gut bacteria can impact how someone responds to therapy and this is by no means an all-inclusive list. So, in terms of statin induced myopathy, let's revisit the ACC/AHA guidelines and see what they list in terms of the predisposing factors. [Fig. 3] They list age, female sex, low body mass index, interacting drugs, comorbidities, and most important to this session, they list agent ancestry is found to have an association. In addition, the FDA actually advises that rosuvastatin be initiated at a lower dose in Asian patients. And

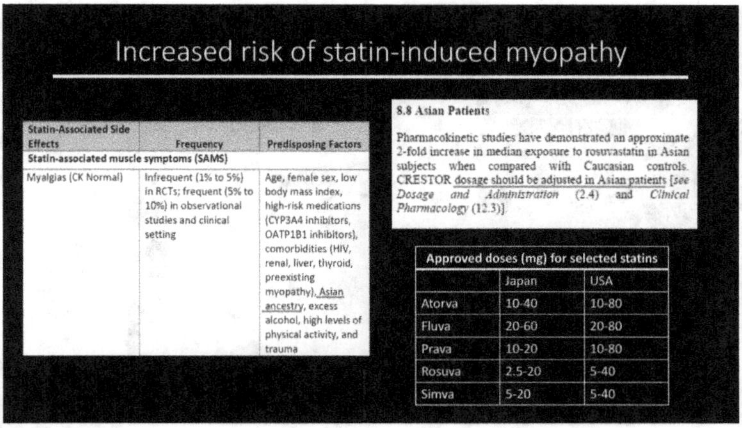

Fig. 3

in Japan, there are no statins that are approved at the highest doses that are approved in the United States.

So let's investigate that a little bit further. [Fig. 4] In this study, they had about 35 individuals in each of these four groups, and they all were given a single dose of rosuvastatin. And then they looked at the pharmacokinetics, or how the drug levels over time, of rosuvastatin. All of these individuals were residents of Singapore, so they're all in the same general location. And they ultimately found about a double of rosuvastatin plasma exposure in these populations, compared to white. So they tried to look for some of the contributing factors and they actually did not find any major factors that contributed. They measured gross dietary intake, they did look at the SLCO1B1 genotype, they all live in Singapore as I mentioned, they also looked at body weight. So it's still unknown whether genetic factors beyond

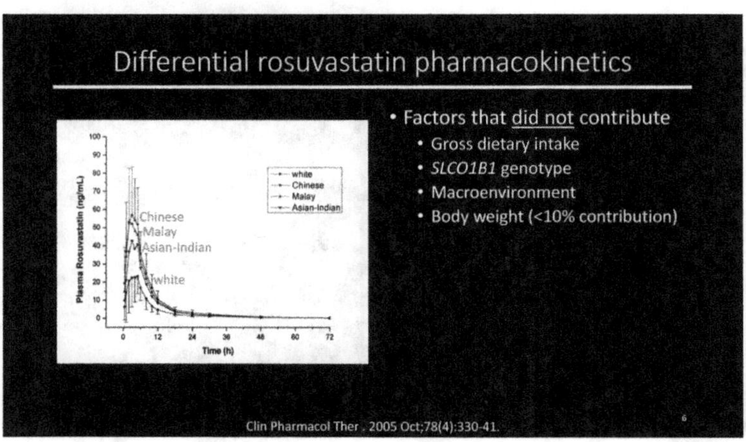

Fig. 4

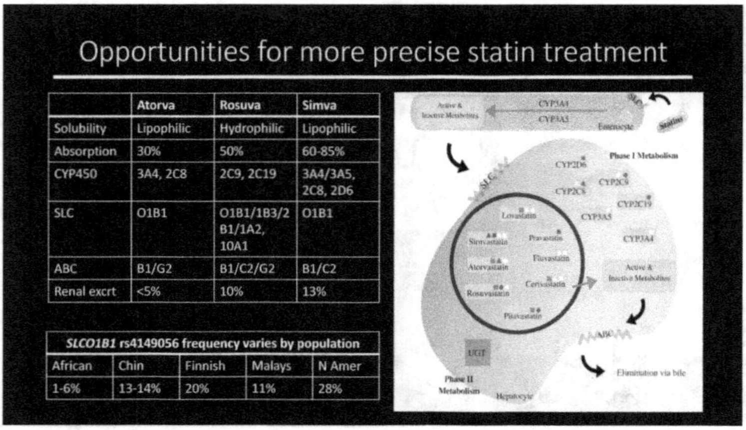

Fig. 5

SLCO1B1 or our social determinants, non-genetic factors are contribute to these differences that they observed.

There are several different statin types, and all the statin types have different biochemical properties. And this influences how the different types are metabolized, and how they are distributed throughout the body. [Fig. 5] And this is further complicated by the findings that the frequencies of the polymorphisms in these various genes within these pathways vary by population. And this is just an example in SLCO1B1. Of course, also, social determinants, as I mentioned, play a huge role here. And so, these all have potential clinical significance. However, there are a lot of gaps in the literature. So ultimately, we need more data with more social determinants, with more genetic variants as covariates, so that we can identify the key contributors to

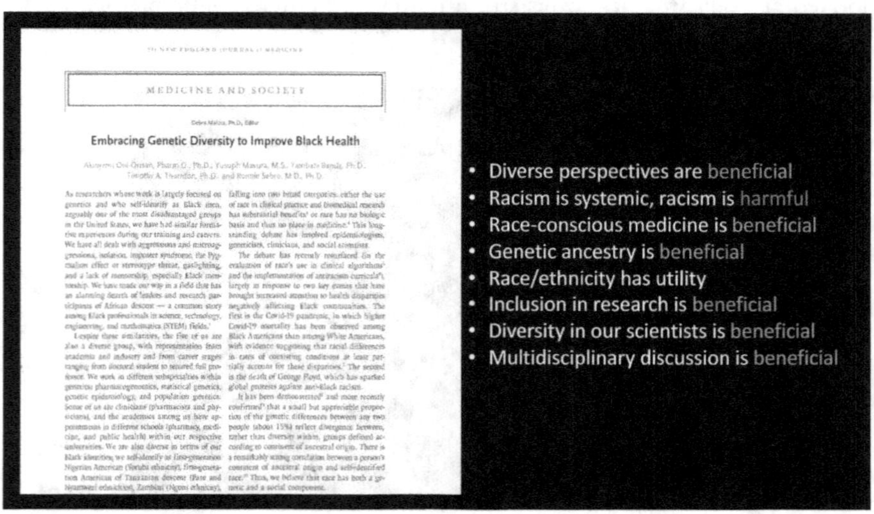

these disparities. And if we can fully characterize the genetic factors and the non-genetic factors that contribute, ultimately race, ethnicity, ancestry are really not necessary if we can determine the functional variants, and the key factors that contribute to this response. But importantly, we need to do this in broad populations.

So, this discussion about the need for inclusion of broad populations perfectly segues into a paper that myself and colleagues recently published, that largely talks about inclusion. [Fig. 6] I wanted to just briefly touch on some of the main themes of the paper. This was a perspective from five Black geneticists, which we thought was a viewpoint that was largely missing in the literature concerning this topic. There actually might only be no more than 10 to 15 Black population geneticists in this in the country, really.

So we talked about racism, we discussed our own experiences as underrepresented minorities in academia, and some of the shared struggles that we experienced. We also talked about COVID-19 disparities in vulnerable communities and these are all under the umbrella of structural racism. We talked about some of the consequences of ignoring race in medicine. And we also delve into the importance of genetic ancestry to ensure that we can capture all of human genetic diversity. We did discuss the utility of race/ethnicity, and how it can help to advance scientific discovery, really as it pertains to ensuring that genetic and clinical research is inclusive and that the results benefit everyone. We also talked about the need for diversity among scientists and clinicians, as well as the benefits of crosstalk between disciplines. So, if these themes resonate with you, for the most part, I would say we're on the same team.

So just to summarize, both genetic and non-genetic factors contribute to drug response. Pharmacogenetics do consider non-genetic factors. We do consider adherence. Adherence and pharmacogenetics can coexist. And it's really important that we consider all factors in order to determine the causal effects of some of the genetic variants. Genetic variation, not race, is the foundation of pharmacogenetics. And, race-based medicine is not the foundation of pharmacogenetics. And finally, implementation of pharmacogenetics in individuals has implications for addressing health disparities at the population level. Thank you.

Moderated Discussion with Flash Talk Speakers

KIRSTEN BIBBINS-DOMINGO: Thank you very much. I'm going to invite all of the speakers for discussion. Thank you for those really outstanding talks. We've had some great questions from the audience and so here's the way I heard your talks. I liked the way that you deconstructed the way we got here and the challenges of using race in our factors. And I'll focus first on Dr. Fontil and Dr. Albert. My question is, both of you have urged us to consider social determinants. I'm going to guess, Valy, when you talk about the low renin levels, that there's probably some evidence, and maybe you can comment on this, [as to] whether social determinants might actually be a grouping that's associated with lower renin levels. In your view, if we measured more social determinants, would we still have race in the way we think about either risk assessment or prescribing because there is a biology of racism? Or do you think that that the that the broader constructs of social determinants then replaces what we have with race in our calculators?

VALY FONTIL: Thanks, Kirsten. The short answer is, I don't know. The short answer is, I think your question is a good study question. I would love to research that. To comment on the first part of your question about renin and how social determinants might contribute to that: It's true, I think that if you look at the levels in renin activity and renin concentration in Black patients, it's low renin, but high pre renin, which tends to indicate that this is at least sort of volume status, sodium retention and volume expansion is probably the main contributing factor to this low renin. And so, clearly, just logically speaking, if you think about allostatic load or psychosocial stress, one of the main things is cortisol level, which would increase sodium retention and volume expansion, which would then cause a low renin. So it definitely stands to reason that these types of social determinants and psychosocial stress would contribute to these differences in biomarker concentrations that we see here.

I should also mention that there are genetic studies about that, that link some polymorphisms to renin levels and into RAS (renin angiotension system). It's kind of beyond my scope of competence. I think there's some complexities in some of these studies, I'm not sure are really good. But they do exist. And some of these polymorphisms are more common in Africa, or people with African ancestry. The problem with that, though, is that there's a wide variety, even just based on geographic variation in Africa itself. So these genes they vary by geographic location in Africa, and there are also other genetic polymorphisms that exist in other ways that are associated with renin level and RAS systems. And so that's why I think the question is somewhat still open in that, if you did adjust for and account for the social determinants, would there still be a remnant sort of genetic related effect or difference based on genetic variation? Maybe, but would it track by race? I don't know. If I had to hypothesize, I might say, maybe not. But I don't know.

KIRSTEN BIBBINS-DOMINGO: Dr. Albert, what do you think? You talked a lot about racism-related biology. There are ways in which we could imagine these might imply innate genetic factors. How would you think, is there still a role if we could measure these things more precisely? Is there a role for self-identified race?

MICHELLE ALBERT: So thanks for a question, Kirsten. I have two approaches to that. The first is that we know that self-identified race does capture factors that are related to racism. Which is why I presented that model of racism-derived stress and the resultant diseases that can occur from them. My approach to the answer to the question about the social determinants and whether or not they would replace race, I think you have to think about it in the structure of surrogate biomarkers, because what we're thinking of is social determinants as a surrogate biomarker for an endpoint.

And there are three things that you have to think about in that context. And let's think about social determinants and race in this. You must have analytic validation, which is relates to reliability of the marker. You must have quantification, which relates to the strength of the marker and the strength that that marker is associated along the pathway of the disease that you're measuring. And that might vary, depending. The influence of the marker may vary on where you are in stage of the disease process. And then you also have to think about utilization, that is the context in which the marker is useful. So let's think about race. If you think of those three things, you know, race doesn't work for validation, it doesn't work for quantification, it doesn't work for utilization. So as a surrogate biomarker, not.

Okay. As we think about the social determinants of health, we need work along these lines. I would suggest that, the validation part of it may be a little bit dicey, the quantification part is possible, and the utilization part is going to be a little bit dicey as well. And so the bottom line is that we need research using broad population samples that are clinical trials, in addition to our epi research, that look at outcomes that incorporate social determinants of health. Sorry for the long answer, but it is intended to be a structural answer.

KIRSTEN BIBBINS-DOMINGO: Excellent, thank you. Now, Dr. Oni-Orisan, you've laid out nicely, and we all know that there are differences in response to therapeutics, help me understand where we are in our knowledge spectrum. Is pharmacogenomics ready for clinical primetime? And what are the dangers of understanding differences by ancestry? Is that a step along the way to actually understanding the basis for the differential drug response? And one of the questions from the audience is, in our highly admixed populations, how do I understand how ancestry that you're studying and helping to elucidate in these differential drug responses? How do I apply that to an individual patient who comes with multiple types of ancestry?

AKINYEMI ONI-ORISAN: Well, I first want to stress that one of the key points of my slides was that genetic variation, the genetic variant itself, is the foundation of pharmacogenetics and how that impacts drug response. So, there's nothing in any pharmacogenomic guidelines about optimizing treatment based on anyone's race or ancestry. So I want to start with that. However, there is utility that Dr. Albert alluded to, of research and brought populations that capture genetic diversity with different ancestries. And race has a utility in terms of capturing that because many individuals don't know their ancestry. So in terms of an admixed individual who I'm seeing as a pharmacologist, providing pharmaceutical care, and recommending optimized therapy for that individual, I wouldn't use any aspect of their ancestry in guiding treatment. However, I would make sure that the literature has individuals that include their ancestry, in order to ensure that they are adequately represented in the studies that ultimately I will use to guide treatment.

In terms of your question about primetime for pharmacogenetics, it depends. I mean, there are specific disease, state specific gene drugs that have adequate evidence that have analytical validity, clinical validity, and clinical utility. And they've shown it in randomized control trials, that it actually reduces costs, it improves safety, and it improves efficacy. CYP2C19, clopidogrel, is an example of a therapy or a genetic test that has been shown to reduce the risk of bleeding, and to reduce the risk of a poor response to completing your treatment in some individuals.

KIRSTEN BIBBINS-DOMINGO: To push a little bit more, though, you are saying that ancestry now is a tool that might help us in discovering the specific variants that would explain differential response, but they would not be how you would implement them clinically.

AKINYEMI ONI-ORISAN: Exactly. So we know that some of the genetic variants differ by population. So we need to make sure we have broad populations in our research.

KIRSTEN BIBBINS-DOMINGO: But we do have, you show in the statin studies, a suggestion that we would choose a different statin based on someone's Asian ancestry.

AKINYEMI ONI-ORISAN: I didn't – I didn't show that.

KIRSTEN BIBBINS-DOMINGO: Is that true or not?

AKINYEMI ONI-ORISAN: So that was recommended by the ACC/AHA guidelines based on the data that I showed. But as I mentioned, they didn't actually determine any of the factors that were contributing to that response. So, basically what I was saying was that more research is needed.

KIRSTEN BIBBINS-DOMINGO: So I'd love each of you to think about this. Because I'm hearing we need more data in how we think about the care for an individual patient, and we need more data in our research across these multiple domains. To go back to the case – each of you are clinicians, each of you practice clinically – what are the dangers of communicating? You're the clinician communicating with Mr. Thomas there, who as you pick up the calculators says Black race differential thing, you chose a different medication, you've suggested that maybe he's going to respond differently. How do we communicate that to patients if you think there's some utility of having these guidelines the way they are now?

MICHELLE ALBERT: I think, Kirsten, it's important – and I have on that slide –how do we know the risks based on the current PCE, based on male, female, Black, white – certainly, there are not similar data for Hispanics or Asians, at this juncture. I think that it is important to tell our patients what we know and what we don't know. And that, medicine, just like anything else, is an evolution over time. We developed antibiotics, after a while of having infections and studying infections. So I think we just have to meet our patients where they are, tell them what we know, and what we don't know. Tell them you know what the current recommendations are and the current potential harms are related to instrumenting a particular therapy. And that is why this needs to be a shared decision making between Mr. Thomas and Dr. Jones, or

Mr. Thomas and Dr. Albert. And I think that fundamentally, it's developing that trust, understanding, who the person is, where they are, what are the influences related. Like where do they live? What are their current stressors that bring that into our clinical therapeutic relationship, and ultimately, are management and it is an evolution that we are in at this point in time.

KIRSTEN BIBBINS-DOMINGO: Great. Dr. Fontil?

VALY FONTIL: I struggle with communication when it comes to the ASCVD risk. I don't think I've ever communicated that to my patients, frankly, as an individual provider. And I think it's harder. I think it's harder with ASCVD risk, because this is a risk score, and then you'd have to tell them why their risk is higher. And I don't know how many clinicians are thinking to tell the patients that other than just calculating the risk and deciding whether to give them statin or not. And to that, I do think that it's important to really make that -- since risk score is a predictive model, then [it] is really important that the model continue to improve to have enough discrimination to be valid enough and not, and not use it inappropriately or an imperfect proxy. And so, I think that is one of the common thing that I see with ASCVD risk and what I see with the evidence in hypertension, is that it's really important to flesh out those these risk models. And so you might see a difference by race, but then what else, understanding what else goes into that. And hypertension, I think I've come to the conclusion that with the ACE inhibitor, as I mentioned, it's really about thinking about how we use ACE inhibitors and when they are appropriate and inappropriate. I've come to the conclusion that we don't need to consider race and that we know enough that it shouldn't be based on race. So, I don't see that as a conversation. It's not as difficult to have that conversation, because I won't bring race into making that decision. Essentially, I'm not going to start an ACE inhibitor monotherapy in most patients regardless of their race.

KIRSTEN BIBBINS-DOMINGO: Dr. Oni-Orisan?

AKINYEMI ONI-ORISAN: I agree with Doctors Albert and Fontil. I guess the one thing I went ahead in terms of communicating to patients that actually helps [is] to have a diverse body of clinicians and scientists to help to communicate with different populations. It helps to have cultural competency. And so we need to start thinking about how we talk about different fields. So that in terms of helping to ensure that we have minority trainees and students going into different fields, and both have scientists and research and clinicians in practice. I don't know too many other Black scientists that do pharmacogenetics, honestly. And, there's been a lot of papers and talks that kind of downplayed some of the importance of fields such as pharmacogenetics. And when you do it in the context of race, it makes it a barrier to get some diverse scientists that want to enter the field. I think, Dr. Kemi Doll wrote a paper in *New England [Journal of Medicine]*, about subspecialties. I think it was called [Structural Solutions for] The Rarest of the Rare, and it was about how it's very difficult to get minorities in some of these subspecialties. So I think that that's really important in communication.

KIRSTEN BIBBINS-DOMINGO: Excellent. Well, thank you so much for your outstanding talks and perspectives. And I think you have given us all a lot to think about. There are some outstanding questions in the chat, and so I think they will help us to continue the discussion in the subsequent panels. But really appreciate you laying out many of the issues on that on a complex topic. Thank you so much.

Moderated Discussion with Responder Panelists

KIRSTEN BIBBINS-DOMINGO: We're going to move now into a commentary and responder panel. I'm pleased to welcome my colleague, Professor Obasogie from the University of California, Berkeley, who has written extensively on the topic of race and medicine. And following his commentary, he will moderate a panel of my colleagues at UCSF: Dr. Denise Connor in the Department of Medicine, who's the leader of our anti-oppression curriculum in the UCSF School of Medicine, Dr. Tung Nguyen, a Professor of Medicine at UCSF who is one of our leaders in diversifying our clinical studies, Dr. Neeta Thakur, who is Professor of Medicine and a pulmonologist who studies factors, both related to environmental, social and dietetic factors related to differential drug response and asthma response and Dr. Teresa Villela, who is the Vice Chair of the Department of Family and Community Medicine, so I will first turn it over to Professor Obasogie.

OSAGIE OBASOGIE: Thank you so much for that introduction. Over the past several months, I've been pleasantly surprised by the number of medical schools and schools of public health that have made clear statements in support of racial minorities in light of the devastating acts of violence we've seen against communities of color. A number of these schools have declared themselves to be anti-racist institutions, or, at the very least, they have stated an aspiration to include anti-racism in their curriculum and activities. So this has been an important gesture. But it's also important to ask whether this is enough.

Anti-racism as an ideal focuses on the individual. It seeks individual training and transformation in how people view the world and how they treat others. To be clear, this is good and necessary work. But as we look at the problem of race in medicine, addressing individual pathologies is not enough. Race is a structural problem in how medicine is organized. So this structural problem is what allows clinicians to assume that Black people feel less pain, and therefore are in less need of pain management options. It's a structural problem that can lead *JAMA* to declare in a tweet that "no physician is racist," and to do so while pretending to explore structural racism itself.

It's also a structural problem that medical schools are producing so few Black and Latinx physicians. Race and racism had been foundational to how medicine has operated for decades, and this new emphasis on individual training on anti-racism often misses this structural dynamic. Put differently, centering the conversation on training individuals to be anti-racist without addressing broader institutional dynamics of race and racism in medicine is not a substantive or meaningful engagement with the problem, and it risks simply turning into another form of public relations.

So as we transition to the next panel, I would like for us to think about ways for clinicians to not only embrace anti-racism in their work, but to develop interventions that can change the way that we do medicine so that we can serve and improve the health of diverse communities. Today we have four esteemed panelists who can help us do this.

First, we have Denise Connor, who's an Associate Clinical Professor at UCSF; we have Tung Nguyen, who is Steven J. McPhee Endowed Chair in General Internal Medicine at UCSF; we have Neeta Thakur, who is an Assistant Adjunct Professor at UCSF; and we have Teresa Villela, who is a Professor of Family and Community Medicine.

I want to start off by asking each of the panelists to talk for a few minutes on their reflections on the previous panel and provide some of their thoughts. And then we'll have some individual questions for the panelists and then open things up to the audience. So first, Denise, do you want to share your initial thoughts or reactions to the first panel discussion?

DENISE CONNOR: Thank you so much. And thank you for your comments and framing of this discussion. I'm very honored to be here with all of you. I actually wanted to address something you were just discussing, which was the structural changes that are needed. And I wanted to make an argument that medical education is a lever for structural change in this realm. And a really important one, certainly not the only one.

When I was listening to the initial case of Mr. Thomas, we heard his voice silenced throughout that encounter. He had many moments where he wanted to ask questions, where he had concerns, and we heard his internal monologue sort of silencing that voice. And when I see that, what I think about is something called *health related stereotype threat*. This is something that one of your colleagues at Berkeley, Dr. Tina Sacks, has written about in a book called *Invisible Visits*. And the idea here is that patients are well aware of the racist history of medicine. They come into the clinical encounter aware of these stereotypes, and many patients spend a lot of emotional and cognitive energy trying to combat those stereotypes. And sometimes that means being silent and not asking questions when they actually have questions, as we saw in this video. And the reason I bring this up, and how this relates to medical education is that, we have a medical education system that is rigidly hierarchical, and that does not necessarily always encourage students to ask critical questions and to be treated as sort of co-learners, especially in the realm of race and racism and medicine.

When they've gone through this training that is very hierarchical and arrive in the clinical setting, they're not really ready to flatten hierarchy in the clinical setting, which is what is needed to let patients break out of the experience of stereotype threat. Patients need to be able to feel centered in the clinical encounter and to feel their voices lifted up. And if we want students to come out of training and be ready to do that, they need to have experienced that throughout their education. So, I would say that bringing an anti-oppressive lens to pedagogy, and the approach that we take for medical education and practicing those principles throughout education will result in students who are ready to be clinicians who can actually enact that kind of approach in the clinical setting as well. I think there's a sort of a structural change to how we teach that has a direct impact, hopefully, on our patients in the future.

OSAGIE OBASOGIE: Great. Thank you so much. Tung, do you want to share some of your thoughts?

TUNG NGUYEN: Yes, thank you. That was a pretty amazing set of presentations. And in particular, I was very appreciative of the complexities and the nuances, and particularly the humility that we just don't know enough. I think the idea is that we're in the middle of a transition time. And the question is, what are the decisions that we're making during transitional period that's going to help us learn more, and come up with better measures or better ways of doing things? And we have to acknowledge this, because I think sometimes … one of my favorite sayings is that there are no simple solutions to complex problems, and the more simplified we try to make it, the worse we make the problem. And that, I think, speaks to your idea about structural issues.

I think biomedicine has always been very reductionistic. I mean, that's the way we do our research. We like to narrow everything down to the single isolatable factor. And then we never, ever get back to opening it up again, to living in a community in this society. And that I think is a fundamental biomedical problem. And the more we focus this conversation between race and biology, we do learn a lot, but then I fear that we never get back to opening it up to how this impacts patients. How does this impact society? How does this impact disparities and equity? And so, I'm glad that we're engaging in this conversation. I don't have an answer. But thanks for having me.

OSAGIE OBASOGIE: Great, thank you. Neeta, would you like to share your thoughts on the first panel?

NEETA THAKUR: Yeah, thank you for having me here today. It's been a really great discussion this morning. I wanted to focus in on a couple of points that were brought up by the case, but then also importantly by the panelists. And I think the first point was that it's really important to think about diversity in research trials. That allows us to examine for differences, not just across population groups, but also to understand what might be contributing to those differences. And I think, in the past, unfortunately, we have applied the differences that we see across socially ascribed racial and ethnic groups directly into clinical practice without often giving consideration to why those differences might be occurring.

I think that clopidogrel is a great example of where the difference may be coming from a genetic variants that may have increased frequency in certain populations. And this actually has something that's really personal to me as someone that's South Asian, and in fact has a nonfunctional CYP2C19 gene and has a family history of heart disease. And so for me that actually has important relevance. But I think we forget to think about, or forget to study, what are those social and environmental contributors that might be contributing to the differences that we're seeing across populations. And I would argue that these structural determinants are probably a larger driver than many of the genetic things that are maybe associated or having found effects in different populations. And so I think this really calls for a big structural change in how we think about funding research and how we support different groups to be able to participate in research and how we think about inviting community to be equal partners in research as we move forward. It would be great to have more support around that piece of it.

OSAGIE OBASOGIE: Great, thank you. And Teresa, would you like to share your thoughts on the first panel?

TERESA VILLELA: Well, huge gratitude for including me in this discussion. I've learned so much already this morning. Let me start by telling you about my favorite pharmacy teacher in medical school all of 30 years ago. He was my favorite because I was fascinated by his area of study. He was a physician scientist, and he studied beta blockers. And remember, this is 30 years ago, so we're talking about Atenolol and Propranolol. So, that was fascinating. But he was also at the end of his discussion, whatever the drug he was telling us about, the physiology, he always ended by saying, "what is a doctor to do?" acknowledging at the end of each session that there are desired effects of our treatments with undesired effects of our treatments, and to be able to be cognizant of both. And then to say, there's so much uncertainty.

And as physicians, as clinicians, we are expected to carry that with us and to bring that with us, not just to clinical encounters, but in the ways in which we organize our practices. So borrowing from that, I think that the next point I'd like to make in response to the wonderful presentations this morning, is to challenge us to think of medicine as a social science. There's a lot of biomedical science that we need to learn from. The social sciences are where our heart is as, again, practicing clinicians, and how we organize our practices and how we organize the delivery of health care. I'll provide a couple of examples, and then we can move on and may be able to cover some of it in more detail.

The first is that we know very well that race concordance and language concordance leads to improved clinical effectiveness. Now what's a doctor to do? And I'm both a clinician educator as well as a clinician administrator. Well, that means that we do really need to challenge ourselves to hire more African American, Black, Indigenous, Asian American clinicians into our practices. Not just into the practice of medicine, but into pharmacy and into an into nurse practitioner school, because this is the way that we will actually begin to change some of the structures that you very well described. Dr. Obasogie.

And I would like to… how much is enough? Justice Ruth Bader Ginsburg was asked often, when are there going to be enough women on the Supreme Court? And she would say, when there are nine. And, of course, people would be shocked. And she would respond by saying, well, there used to be nine men, and nobody ever raised a question about that. So that's one area that I would bring to you for consideration. We also see better adherence, better results, more effectiveness in our clinical practice, when our patients trust us. And how do we build that trust?

Well, one way is by not being the all-knowing, shake your finger, you got to do this sort of clinician, but also working in collaboration. Again, with clinical pharmacists, with other clinicians, with health coaches, who have to be at the place that our patients come to, with their questions related to their medical treatment, but also with their uncertainties about all of the things that that make their lived experience that is thought of as outside of healthcare practice. I think when we do that, and when we do it over time, not just one clinical encounter, or three clinical encounters over a year period, but truly over decades. And again, that's why it cannot only be me, but it has to be the collaborators that I have in my clinical practice, when you build that trust, over 10 years, over a generation, so that when a parent brings their child, that child brings their friend when they're a teenager, because they trust you to treat them in a respectful manner, then that actually begins to make some changes. Thank you.

OSAGIE OBASOGIE: Great, thank you so much. So I'm going to pose a couple of questions to our panelists. And then we're going to shift over to some questions from the audience. So please, if you have questions for the panelists, please submit them to the Q&A button and we'll start reviewing those questions shortly.

My first question is for Denise. So in your opening remarks, you talked a bit about medical education, and your work in that area. And I was wondering if you could talk more about where medical education has been and where it's going with regards to the use of race in medicine? I would really like to hear you expound upon that a little bit.

DENISE CONNOR: Thank you so much for that question. I think there's a lot to say here. I'm going to focus in a little bit on the hidden curriculum as a way for us to think about this. I think a lot of what we teach is implicitly taught when it comes to race and racism, and has deeply powerful and harmful impacts that have been perpetuated in medical education for a very long time. When you think about the hidden curriculum, I think looking at how we present patient cases, throughout medical school is a really illustrative example.

For a long, long time, there were many explicit racist ways that patients were being discussed in clinical cases throughout medical school. And a number of years ago we recognized that and were horrified. And the response was, let's take race out of all of the critical cases. Let's have this sort of colorblind approach to how we teach and that will solve the problem.

While that was certainly well meaning. We talk about impact versus intention – the impact was not what was intended. The impact was, we first of all centered white patients. And because we're sort of in a sea of white supremacy, when race was not mentioned, students assumed we were talking about white patients as the default. And that was very problematic. There were certain assumptions that were being communicated without actually saying anything. And then when race was mentioned, because race wasn't completely taken out, there was this idea that when it was "clinically relevant," we could include race. And what that did was, in the minority of times when we mentioned race, provide very stereotypical ways that that was brought up.

And there was this implicit belief that there were certain diseases that were, for example, Black diseases. And if you know them, then that's what you should think about when you see a Black patient. Otherwise, we're talking about the default white patient. And that propagated these sort of false notions of race as biology and buttressed these ideas that race is fundamentally a biologic thing, when in fact, we certainly know that is not true and is a very harmful, harmful thing.

Well, certainly racism, as was mentioned by Dr. Albert, can become biology, race itself, as we've been discussing, is a social and political construct. And so being able to tease those things out is important. When I think about where do we go from here, to put people's full social context back into medical education, which is I think where we need to go, I think the important thing to think about is being willing to be transparent with our students about what we know and what we don't know. So engaging students around when we're bringing up race in this case, why are we doing that? Let's disambiguate the many different ways that that might be interpreted so that people aren't leaving a session with false ideas about what was meant when race was brought up.

If we are talking about a study that involves race, were the authors able to actually say what race was being used as a proxy for? Is that clear? Or is that not clear? Was this good science? Or was this not good science? Is race an appropriate proxy in that in that setting? Being able to have those conversations is important. And then being able to recognize the impact of social determinants of health and racism, experiences of racism and being able to be clear about why are we talking about race. What are the limits of our understanding in a given situation, when we are talking about race so that students aren't leaving with sort of these misconceptions about how it is relevant in a given situation? I think that's really important. And I also think it hopefully will lead students to be able to have that critical mindset, when they go out and talk in the clinical setting or read papers, where race is being described, they'll be in the habit of asking these critical questions. Are we in a trap of sort of thinking about correlation as causality? Is race actually the right thing to be measuring here? Is this an appropriate proxy? What do we want to measure? And sort of pushing us forward to ask these really challenging questions and to dive into the complexity that we are in when we talk about these issues?

OSAGIE OBASOGIE: Great, thank you so much. So my next question is for Tung. We have spent a lot of time in this panel, encouraging all of us to think beyond biology when conceptualizing race, and I want to ask you, are there potential complications or downside to having this conversation about race beyond kind of biology or genetics be a determinant way of thinking about health outcomes?

TUNG NGUYEN: Thanks, Osagie. Yes, I do think this is a necessary conversation. In these kinds of controversial conversations, semantics are used both unconsciously and consciously to move the conversation forward. And they have effects that I think sometimes go beyond what we think. So this whole statement that race is not biology, I worry. I worry because it's stripped of context. And I think for a lot of us who do social work, social related work with medicine, I want us to say race is not biology and biology is not health. Because if we do that, then we understand that we're not stripping … the primacy of our system is on biology. We think about health as disease oriented. We think about biology as the key determinant of disease and health. And we fund that way, we teach that way, we take care of patients that way, many times, consciously or unconsciously. And when we deemphasize race … When we say race is not biology, even though we are well meaning, I think we're deemphasizing race, which I actually worry about. We don't want to erase race because it matters so much in so many different ways. And so I want us to think about the implications of what we're doing when we do that. That's really the main sort of worry that I have.

OSAGIE OBASOGIE: So thank you, that that really connects nicely with Teresa's previous comments about how medicine is a social science. And I think that's a really important way of thinking about the social and the political in shaping health outcomes. I want to turn next to you, Teresa. So how can we ensure that patients and communities voices are heard and prioritized when making decisions about how race is used in medicine? Do you have any thoughts on that?

TERESA VILLELA: Thank you. Yes. Again, these are not new ideas. We're talking about the 1970s. Clinics Without Walls. Do any of you remember? Clinics without walls -- What does that mean? It means that really, the neighborhood is the clinic. I think this is important in the context that we're talking about, aside from the racialized ways in which Black African American individuals and families and communities suffer in this country, aside from police violence, redlining, food insecurity, inadequate housing, environmental racism, discriminatory hiring practices, which were all mentioned at the beginning of the video, there's also economic segregation.

So segregation through economic wealth, but then also in employment as it has been so clarified by the COVID-19 epidemic in who has fallen due to that. And then education segregation: segregation of high-quality education in this country is rampant. And so why is neighborhood health important? Why should there be clinics without walls, hospitals without walls, that may be taking it a little too far. But the idea is [to be] health centered, because health is not only the absence of disease, but being health centered brings in the voices of the folks that we're trying to care for. And we're reinventing that; we've started to reinvent that in the last, I would say, five to 10 years, bringing in patient advisory councils, into clinics, into public health centers, but also into privately held health centers, into medical institutions. And so I think that that begins to get at that. We can't only bring their voices, though, we also need to bring their agency for them not only to be able to say to us, this needs to be done differently, but when they say, actually, *this is a better way*, this is a better idea. This is something that needs to be tried to have a way for that to have the right amount of power, so that we don't take 20 years again, to come back to learning the same lesson and having to reestablish community engagement and community trust all over again.

OSAGIE OBASOGIE: Great, thank you so much. And Neeta, during our first session, one of the keynote speakers, Dr. Burchard, describes some of the biological and genetic predispositions that lead to poor health outcomes in minority communities with regards to asthma and other respiratory problems. So, many see this as a controversial perspective on health disparities regarding pulmonary function, and outcomes are deeply entwined with social, political, environmental, and political factors. So, I'm wondering if you could talk more about these contextual factors, and how they might call into question some of the genetic explanations for health disparities in lung functioning?

NEETA THAKUR: Thank you for that question. I think when we talk about lung function specifically, it's important to reflect that there are many determinants of lung function, and one of the largest contributors just how tall you are. So individuals that are taller have larger lung function. We also have really good evidence that there are certain exposures that are particularly toxic to the lung. So tobacco smoke being the most well supported one, whether that's *in utero*, over the childhood, or as a smoker yourself, there's a direct effect on how big your lungs will eventually become over childhood and early adulthood and then also an accelerated effect on lung function as you age.

We also have good evidence that where you live, what you experience and your socioeconomic position has impact on lung function. One of the largest and greatest body of evidence is for environmental exposures, with one of the best studies coming out of USC with the Children's Health Study. That group not only showed that poor air quality was associated with decreased lung function in children, they also showed through a really nicely use of a natural experiment design, that when with EPA regulation and improvement in air quality, we actually saw lung function improve in children. So showing this direct effect, if you take away the toxin, you can actually see improvement in a very short period of time.

And so, given that these social and environmental determinants are strongly influenced by which racial or ethnic group you are a part of, in that historic and current practices not only dictated where individuals were allowed to live, but also the resources that were invested or, in fact not invested in those communities, I think it's really important to acknowledge that the lower lung function values that we are observing and these large population studies comparing Black populations with non-Hispanic white groups that these factors, these contextual factors are likely being reflected in this overall need deficit. And by using population norms and race specific equation, we may actually be missing this pathology. I don't want to suggest that like that there isn't a role for genetic factors or, you know, sometimes in some instances, they can have a strong influence. But I think compared to the overall contribution of these contextual factors that are more difficult and nuanced to measure because we haven't applied the same statistical methods, or like the funding on being able to measure factors that occur over a life course and sometimes over generations, we just haven't gotten there with the science to sort of prove this. But I do think that there is a strong component for contextual factors.

OSAGIE OBASOGIE: Great, so thank you so much. I'm now going to turn things over to Aimee Medeiros, who's an Associate Professor of History and Health Sciences at UCSF. And she's going to assist with bringing forth a few questions from the audience.

AIMEE MEDEIROS: Thank you. Okay, I have a question that is meant for each panelist. This person would like to ask each panelist whether they as clinicians would use the ASCVD calculator with the race variable included when seeing Mr. Thomas, and if so, what they would say to Mr. Thomas, about the basis of his risk estimation. I can call on someone. Perhaps Dr. Connor, would you like to begin?

DENISE CONNOR: Thanks, Aimee. That's a really important question. From what we talked about, I feel like we've all kind of skirted this sort of practical, concrete question. So, I appreciate the person who asked it. I think, like I talked about transparency, and not shying away from complexity being important with our students, I think the same is true with our patients. And if we do have a flattened hierarchy in which we can actually have honest, authentic conversations with patients where they can share with us their concerns about how racism impacts their care, for example, and how discrimination has impacted their care. And we can share with them our concerns about how racism impacts medical research, and how things are framed and performed.

I think having a conversation, when we talk about shared decision making, we need to have that background conversation first, to say this score includes race, I think race has been used as the proxy for many different possible things here. And they're not teased out. And I'm not sure you as an individual person, Mr. Thompson, which of these factors you actually possess, I'm not sure. And we need to learn more about you as a person to tease that out.

We saw that great list that Dr. Albert showed, all those different social determinants of health and other factors that may contribute to risk, and being able to sort of talk with the patient about which of those factors he may have to add to what the risk score is telling us, I think is important and treating that person as an individual, taking the time to learn about them. And then also saying, here, these are the numbers, this is what it says if I put Black race in, this is what I get if I don't. We're not sure we understand what that means yet. And let's have a conversation about that. And, sort of being honest about the limits of our knowledge with our patients.

TUNG NGUYEN: I can also take a crack at that. And actually, I don't have an answer. After 30 years of clinical care, the first thing that comes to mind when that question comes up is, oh, my God, you know, I got 20 minutes. Do I really want to open this can of worms, even as big of an important thing as it is. And both in terms of just explaining how race is incorporated into the guideline recommendation, and two, whether or not does that open up a whole discussion about race and racism, that I'm not ready to have with my patient. I will say, though, that *vis a vis* the whole workforce diversity issue, I am much more comfortable having this conversation with an Asian patient than I am with a non-Asian patient. And I think that that's something that as we go forward with figuring out how to do this work, I think we need more diversity in our clinicians, in our clinician educators and our research because that enables us to have these conversation without problem. I will say that, for example, I don't have a problem with bringing up race, like Black race, in the decision to talk about prostate cancer screening. But I do have a problem with sort of these other sort of guidelines. That seems to be much more complicated. So I'll stop there.

KIRSTEN BIBBINS-DOMINGO: Can I step in to answer this. I think the challenge for us is that the use of these risk calculators is for a biomedical decision that is whether we start a statin. And I think the challenge of these calculators, without race, underestimate the true risk of heart attacks that we see in African American communities. It underestimates the true risk of heart disease that we see in poor communities. And then the question is, is statin the treatment for racism or poverty? Well, a statin is not a reasonable treatment for those. But it actually is important that clinicians understand that these are factors that have real health consequences for communities, for poor communities, for our minoritized communities. And so the challenge for how we teach and how we practice is how do you understand what we are observing, what really has these larger structural factors that are at play that Professor Roberts and Professor Obasogie point us to, but then not lead us to this very biomedical decision, well that means they need a higher dose of statins, because that is the treatment that the risk calculator points us to. And I think that's where it's incumbent upon all of us to think of our patients within the broader context, and ourselves within the broader context. And so that's why it's hard. It's not a simplistic answer to that question, because the recognition is still important.

TERESA VILLELA: I use that calculator all the time, because I otherwise have no idea what to do with statin treatment. And I think it's useful in that sense. That's not entirely true, but it gives me a range. It gives me an idea of whether this person in front of me, what their risk may be for cardiovascular disease in the next 10 years. And I completely appreciate what Dr. Bibbins-Domingo is saying about underestimation and taking that into account. Why don't we talk to our patients about it? I learned the most about this from a couple of things. One is that one of our health workers, who has been working with our team in the Family Health Center around improving blood pressure control among African Americans, said to our group once, you know, had this conversation with a patient who, we're trying to bring their blood pressure to control, and it was a difficult conversation and a lot of things going on. And finally I just said to her, you know, the reason that we're health educators or health workers, is a Black woman said to her, the reason that we're focusing on you is because Black individuals in general in our community have very poor control, and found that that created an opening for conversation that was very rich, and that otherwise would not have happened. Now, they were across from each other. And so they knew each other's skin color. But it was more in identifying reason that this is important to me, is because I care about you and I care about our community together.

So that has given me the courage to bring up that conversation more frequently. And I think it has gone very well, I think it has informed me, and I think it's helped to build trust. The other thing that I will say is that Dr. Tony Martin, who is a physician in the East Bay, a primary care physician, wrote an article about use of the GFR equation about 10 years ago, I think it's called the color of kidneys, in which she taught very prominently about the ways in which she thought about these conversations with her patients. She's African American, and many of her patients are as well. And the question that's not being asked is are my kidneys Black. I've always thought of that, … But I think that the ways in which our patients hear our discussion of race, we need to just be really careful and listen to them more, rather than just sort of harming by including language that is just going to make them mistrust us even more.

OSAGIE OBASOGIE: So Tung, one thing you mentioned in your comment is that you would consider prostate cancer guidelines a bit differently. I was wondering if you would like to expand on that?

TUNG NGUYEN: Maybe I didn't really mean that it's biologically different. But it's just so clear. I do a lot of cancer prevention work, and the data on the disparities in prostate cancer and how we think about it, in terms of recommending a PSA or prostate specific antigen test is so complicated. Race does factor into it, at least for now it does. And we have these conversations all the time with our communities.

I don't do a lot of work with Black communities, but our Cancer Center does. And our Black patients that we engage with, the Black community leaders we engaged with, do want to emphasize that yes, being Black puts you at higher risk for prostate cancer. And yes, you should think about prostate cancer screening differently than a white person would. That's the feedback we're getting. And so for me that feels comfortable that I can use that particular way of looking at a race in this particular clinical situation. I do want to say, though, that the point I was making, it's important who is involved in these conversations. Again, I'm very interested in who is the dominant group driving the conversation. And even as a great group as we are here in these conversations, it's still very much academic focus, very scientific knowledge, prioritization. I think communities and the patient's perspective should be a part of this.

NEETA THAKUR: Just to add to what's been discussed already around the use of the algorithm for statin therapies. One piece in thinking about patients with asthma and addressing whether or not we need to increase their treatment versus talk about other sources is when you have someone with high cholesterol or with poor asthma control to try to think about the social or environmental contributors that might be leading to that being out of control and why those might be different for different groups. So housing security, food security, having access to healthy foods and vegetables, access to exercise, both being able to do it safely in your neighborhood, or having the time, sleep-wake cycles.

We know that employment history has an important impact on people having to work at night versus during the day, that has disruption to your ability to manage your lipids. And so, I think when we see that race is being incorporated in these guidelines, we have to really, really reflect and think about what it is actually measuring. And you know, to echo both Kirsten and Tung, these differences that we're seeing in populations should really have us questioning what are they reflecting. And then how do we talk with our patients about this. And so in my own practice, asthma is easy because it is in the guidelines to ask about environmental exposures. I end up doing that early. Day one. In the guidelines, it's recommended to do it only after the person has uncontrolled asthma for some time, and you've already done step up therapy, I think it's a little bit backwards. There's good evidence, if you address environmental and social factors, you can get good asthma control 70% of the time. And so I think the way we talk about the social factors should be the same way we talk about BMI or blood pressure with our patients.

OSAGIE OBASOGIE: Great, thank you. Denise, did you want to add a few comments?

DENISE CONNOR: I just wanted to add one thing. Echoing what Teresa was saying, and something I said earlier about talking with patients about their experiences in healthcare around discrimination and racism, I think it does feel like opening Pandora's box, certainly in a 15-minute visit. But we talk about very complex things with patients. We talk about end-of-life care, we talk about sexual history, we talk about things that are very complicated and challenging to talk about because they're important. And I think we actually need evidence-based approaches to how to open up these conversations with patients about identity and background about experiences in the healthcare system.

I don't think we have all the right language yet. We certainly don't have the training. Denise Davis, which was one of a wonderful faculty member here in the Department of Medicine, has developed some conversation openers to talk to patients about their background and identity and how that's impacted them in their lives in very positive ways in terms of how their resilience and their strengths from their community, as well as potentially in ways that have been challenging in health care setting. I hope to see in the future that we continue to push, what are the right ways to open these conversations and we don't shy away from them, because they're in the room. They're the elephant in the room. Patients come into the healthcare setting worried about this. You know, it's not like we're opening up something that they're not already thinking about many times. So I do think that's important. And I think that's research is needed really to help us do that well.

OSAGIE OBASOGIE: Great, thank you. Aimee, do you have another question from the audience?

AIMEE MEDEIROS: I do. Thank you. This question has to do with the structural and social factors that are sometimes overlooked when we use a reductionist clinical research frame. And this is for the entire panel. Can you please comment on the lack of use of, and support for, social science research in academic medicine that would be better prepared methodologically and theoretically, to understand the social structural factors driving biological responses? How can we change this in the moment of recognition of structural racism and racism over race as causative?

TUNG NGUYEN: I think that we need to spend a lot more money, prioritize research not just on the social determinants of health, but exactly the kind of things that Denise and Teresa are talking about. Like how do we communicate? How do we talk to people? How do we include all of these things in the work that we do? We just don't have enough money. I mean, we can we map the human genome. We're nowhere near where we need to be for this work to happen with an adequate level of scientific precision, I have to say. You know, even like, if, let's say we wanted to replace or moderate the effect of race with racism, do we even know how to measure racism in a way that's validated? Or across populations, things like that, these questions just have not been answered scientifically. And we're not investing in it. We're having this conversation where we're not going to invest in the most important things that are determining health.

NEETA THAKUR: I will just add to that. In addition to thinking about how these structural and social determinants impact health, we also, at the same time, need to think and promote interventions, both at the policy, community, and individual level that actually can change or impact these social and structural determinants in a way to improve health. There has been a large body of research that do show that social and structural determinants, including racism, impacts health, and since I see Dr. Perez-Stable has been able to join us, the NIHD just put out a really nice RFA on the structural determinants of health and putting funding towards it. And part of that RFA is a focus towards interventions. And so, we also need to move beyond describing the problem and start focusing towards interventions both at the policy, community, and individual level that brings in communities as equal partners. And that needs financial support, we can't expect people just like we as researchers are funded to do our job, we need to fund community members in the same way to be part of that conversation and part of directing those research initiatives.

DENISE CONNOR: I was going to add, that when you think about anti-oppression and anti-racism, that includes other ways of knowing, besides traditional, Western, often white ways of knowing. So that includes storytelling, and it includes fields outside of medical education, for sure. So if we're serious when we say we want to bring an anti-oppressive lens to medical education, I think we absolutely need the expertise of people outside of the very narrow biological view of health. As been brought up, health is much more complicated than just biology. And so I don't have an answer to the funding piece or how to really do this, except to say, I completely agree, it's important and if we're serious about moving in this direction, we need to accept that RCTs are not the only type of knowledge that we should be learning from.

OSAGIE OBASOGIE: Just to add to this, from the pedagogical side, I am a faculty member in the Joint Medical Program between UCSF and Berkeley. And that program has been around for about four decades and it was intentionally designed to have a more integrated process in teaching medical students in ways that brings in the social sciences and humanities as a central part of their medical training. So, our students, while they're getting their initial training in both the sciences and clinical trainings, they're also receiving or have the opportunity to explore the health sciences and how social and political and economic factors impact health by being able to spend two and a half years on Berkeley's campus and making those connections within their medical training and in other parts of the university. And it's a phenomenal program. And it's unique.

But still, we have a lot of work to do in making sure that that integration to other social sciences and humanities really speaks in meaningful ways to their clinical training. And so you know, a lot of my work is constantly trying to find ways to make sure that the work that you're doing in my class that puts medicine in this broader historical and social context, making sure that that's meaningful, as a way to inform the way that they interact with patients, or interact whether other physicians as part of their education. So this is to say that, even in a space, like a Joint Medical Program, where I would like to think that we are doing it in the best way, or the most advanced way possible, we still have so much work to do in making sure that we help our students fully understand and appreciate those direct connections between the social sciences and humanities, and the work that they would do as trained physicians. And I think that's something that all of us as educators can continue to work on.

TERESA VILLELA: I couldn't agree more. So I'm going to just add my voice to say yes, yes, and yes. I think that social sciences have scientifically shown us again, and again, how we can contribute to people's health. And we've excluded them, sometimes on purpose, and sometimes unintentionally, from the training of the next generation of healthcare providers. Again, I'm going to just name a couple because I try to have these instruct my day-to-day practice.

One is that we know that structured social learning and learning to learn at the age of three to four has huge and profound and long lasting impacts for social determinants of health and for ameliorating some of the some of the usually called negative social movements. And the second thing is that if we agree that economic segregation is part of the problem that contributes to poor health, then having a guaranteed income is something that has been studied by social scientists over and over again. It's shown in cases where it's tied to an actual health practice, like getting immunizations, it makes a difference. But every single time, it always adds to folks' sense of well-being. So even if we don't meet the metrics, people feel better. They have more agency over their day to day lives. And so that means that they will be healthier. And so, again, I couldn't agree more. And wanted to add that.

OSAGIE OBASOGIE: Any other comments on this question? And if not, we can move on to the next one. Okay, Aimee.

AIMEE MEDEIROS: Another question is actually a couple of them together. And not only from this session, but from the last one. And it has to do with many of our attendees being students. And we get it. We got asked this question last time and this time about what students can do to raise their concerns and ask critical questions about race, racism, education, causes of medical mistrust, and more during classes, and to instructors that these topics are not openly being discussed in the curriculum, and then also, too, in clerkship. So hoping that you would be able to provide some advice for our students who are tuning in today.

DENISE CONNOR: I'm happy to start with that. What I was going to say is that feedback, when done well, is based on relationships, and mutual respect and trust. And so I think the Academy of Communication in Healthcare is a fantastic organization that helps us think about how to talk with people, how to talk with our patients, how to talk with our colleagues. And a really important thing that they have re-coined the phrase feedback to *relationship centered feedback*. So I think that's the first thing I would say, which is that being able to provide constructive feedback or to bring up challenging conversations really requires an investment in other people as humans, and a recognition of your kind of common beliefs and values.

I actually think one thing we've been talking about is, we don't really teach how to provide feedback or how to receive feedback all that often throughout medical education. And it's actually critical to continuing to improve as clinicians and as members of clinical teams. So I think that's something that is needed is actually structured curriculum to help all of us learn better how to do that work. I think in the meantime, the thing that everyone always brings up is humble inquiry, right. Humble inquiry is a helpful kind of thing to keep in mind when you are bringing up challenging questions, which is to say things in the frame of, *I'm curious about this ... I'm noticing that we're using race in this way ... And I'm curious to learn more about it.* It can be a very helpful way to open conversations that does not immediately lead to defensiveness and fragility on the part of people that are receiving those questions. So I think focusing on your shared values and beliefs, the relationships that you have, and then using a frame of humble inquiry is a start. But I think in reality, what we need his actual training of learners as well as faculty how to have these conversations.

TUNG NGUYEN: I want to make a comment. Whenever it's a question that relates to power dynamics, I always want to challenge it. Like why is the onus on the students to learn how to do this better? Every time we present stuff to our senior faculty and our senior researchers, we find that they're incredibly deficient. They don't know how to talk to patients. They don't know how to work with communities. They don't know how to deal with race and disparities and equity. And we somehow give them a pass, and it's on our students learn how to do it. I think we need to hold people accountable. And it goes beyond just DEI training and implicit bias training. Those things are really necessary, but it's just not sufficient. And so when we think about medical education reform in this area, it's about our faculty. I think our teachers are great, and our students are great, but it's the other people who interact with our students on a regular basis are actually driving along this conversation.

OSAGIE OBASOGIE: Tung, I really want to emphasize the point that you've made, because it's so important. One of the conversations that I always hear from faculty is that the race conversation is just too hard. So I'm not going to address it in my class. And I think, as you said, we really need to challenge that point and realize that as university faculty, as researchers, we are engaged in cutting-edge research that is transforming the world, right? So you're a cancer researcher, I do work in law and reproductive genetic technologies, all of us on this panel are doing phenomenal work. We are at institutions, UCSF and Berkeley and other places that are doing critical work. If we can engage in that work, we can engage the race conversation.

And it's one thing for something to be technically difficult. It's another thing for it to be politically difficult. And we need the courage to engage the politically and socially difficult questions, in ways and with a level of seriousness that we address other parts of our research endeavors, because it's so central to what we do. And moreover, when we neglect to address those issues and questions, we are failing our students, we're failing our institutions, and we're failing our communities. So just as it's important for us to build competency in the kind of tested technical skills that we train our students in, so too is it important for us to build competency in the way for our students to be able to engage the world around them, which includes being able to have sophisticated and meaningful and authentic conversations about race and racism. And that's a huge responsibility on us as researchers, scholars and teachers, and it's a huge responsibility for institutions that we work for to take seriously as well. So I think the point that you're making is so critical for us to rethink and reimagine what our responsibilities are in teaching the next generation.

NEETA THAKUR: I want to echo the power dynamics. I do think this needs to come from the top, the leaders, to have this actually translate. I do know and recognize that that's slow and frustrating at the training level. And so, sort of pragmatic suggestions for trainees, understanding that the medical education system is incredibly hierarchical. Your evaluations are dependent on your interactions with your faculty and clinical instructors. There is an overemphasis on being the stereotypical best student when you're on rotation, so questioning practices and decision making is not favored. Humble inquiry is one way. I have seen the power of anonymous feedback, especially when it comes from large numbers of trainees, and also banding together. Remember, UCSF did not make this focus until the medical students formed the White Coats for Black Lives, right? That pushed UCSF to change focus and does the Difference Matters Movement. And so that was coming from our from our students effort. And so I think there is power. I've also seen it happen both at the resident and fellow level as well, where change has happened. The other way to bring it in is through academic discourse. Just like we talked about seminal articles, and RCTs, we should be including in our journal clubs, which are often brought by the students and trainees on those that highlight health disparities, and the social determinants and structural determinants of health and talk about them at the same scholarly level and their implications for clinical practice on a regular basis. And so those are efforts that can be done and more tangible right now, as we wait for this sort of slower process for it to happen from the leaders.

DENISE CONNOR: I do want to quickly just reflect on your point, Tung. Faculty development is a core part of anti-oppression work for sure. I think the key thing, though, is that it is slow. I mean, that's reality. So I think we do need things that you just talked about Neeta, which are what do you do in the meantime, while we're working on up here, as that hopefully begins to change culture, what do students do in the meantime, tomorrow? And I think that's a challenging place to be for students.

TUNG NGUYEN: I have a pitch over this. We don't have a diverse enough Academy. And we've been waiting for the pipeline to fill that lack of diversity and it's taking forever and I'm not really sure that we are all that successful. I mean, at UCSF, I think we are doing a good job. I just feel like we need to introduce more diverse voices into the Academy. I think community engagement, diverse community engagement, particularly of community leaders with life experiences, and as you mentioned, Denise, other kinds of knowledge besides academic, scientific research knowledge into our education system is important. We need to introduce them, we need to reimburse them, we need to prioritize them. We need to treat them as valued teachers just like anybody else.

OSAGIE OBASOGIE: Great. So I believe we are at our time limit. So I want to thank all of our panelists for these extraordinary comments and reflections. This has been, I think, really useful and productive. And I hope to be in conversation with you all in the future. I will turn things back over to Kirsten.

KIRSTEN BIBBINS-DOMINGO: Well, you certainly have an open invitation from us to continue to engage us in these conversations. And we really appreciate both your commentary, Professor Obasogie, and my thanks to all of my colleagues, Dr. Connor, Dr. Villela, Dr. Nguyen, and Dr. Thakur. Thank you very much. We're going to transition to some closing comments from someone who is well known to us at UCSF and now known to the rest of the country, Eliseo Pérez-Stable, who is director of the National Institutes on Minority Health and Health Disparities at the National Institutes of Health, and a general internist and colleague and mentor to many of us at UCSF. We've talked about many of the factors that relate to how we think about the knowledge generation we need in this area. And as one of the largest funders of this type of work at the NIH, we were really pleased that Dr. Pérez-Stable agreed to join us. He's going to give some remarks, and then I will come back and talk with him briefly about this, and then we'll close out the session.

Closing Comments

Eliseo Pérez-Stable, MD

ELISEO PÉREZ-STABLE: Thank you very much. Kirsten. It's wonderful to see old friends. And I do plan to try and join you next week as well for the earlier part of the session. This is always of relevance to, well to everything I do, that's for sure.

So this is the only sort of standard definition slide, just what we use at NIH. [Fig. 1] The populations with health disparities are listed at the first four bullets. I would add that the first three were part of our original legislation in the year 2000. You learn in federal government, you can't change things that are mandated by congressional law. So those are there to live. Just to reiterate, all racial ethnic minorities as defined by the US Census, all poor people of any color, rural residents, and I added the qualifier of underserved when I started in NIMHD. And then in 2016, sexual and gender minorities were added to populations with health disparities with the qualifier of for NIH research purposes.

And we use the operational definition of a health outcome that is worse than one of these populations, usually compared to a reference group as defining a health disparity. Then, we also embrace the notion, I think this was critical in getting over the barriers for sexual and gender minorities, with the department at the time under the Obama administration, that all these populations have a social disadvantage that result in part from being subject to discrimination or racism, and also being underserved in health care.

So it is fundamentally important, in my view, that race/ethnicity is a self-identified social construct. [Fig. 2] That's a given. I don't believe that every NIH leader or Institute director or scientist in their heart of hearts believes that. But at least they don't contradict me in public. I also believe that this complicated

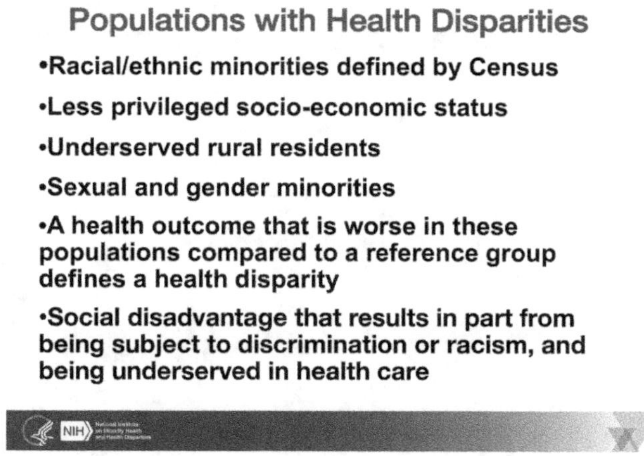

Fig. 1

social construct that we use and operationalize has global implications and is not a US issue, as I was told by colleagues in Latin America 30 years ago. It has behavioral, biological, and environmental components that are important, as well as social interaction components.

Race/ethnicity differences are really a potential tool for discovery science at all levels. And I think it's something that has been sort of at this core of my own research career from the start at a time where I did not have these kinds of concepts at all. However, it's important to embrace the idea that the legacy of racism and discrimination as well as individual experiences really do travel with the self-identified race/ethnicity. So why does this construct explain so much is the question. It's not that race/ethnicity is causing anything. I think that's the wrong way to operationalize it, and people are debating that. It's

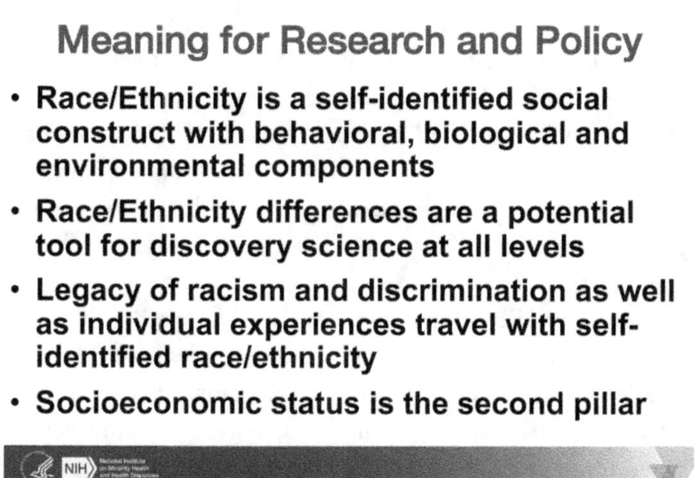

Fig. 2

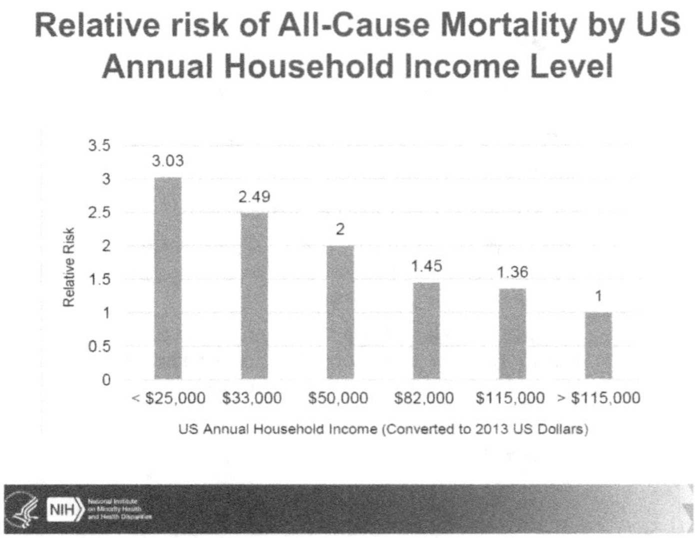

Fig. 3

an association that we observe, and therefore that should lead you to inquiry scientifically, or interventions, or ways to manage either programs or in this case, patients.

I think equally important to consider in this discussion, at all levels, that socioeconomic status or social class, to use the social science terminology, is equally important as self-identified race/ethnicity. And we have really fallen most short in this concept. Many clinical investigators or clinicians either believe they know the race/ethnicity of their patient or ask or in a research context, sometimes people ask, but they very infrequently know or ask about social class. And I think this is a major deficiency that needs more attention. This is a simple way to illustrate the point about the importance of socioeconomic status taken from data from the IRS, used by a number of different economists over the years, Raj Chetty maybe most recently. [Fig. 3] If you're under $25,000 in household income for a family of four, this roughly is the poverty level in the US, roughly about 15% of Americans live there, you're three times more likely to die from anything than if your household income of four is $115,000, which is definitely well off, but you probably still got, or will get, a recovery check coming up, because you qualify. So you're not wealthy is the point.

These predict a lot, I think you're all familiar with this. [Fig. 4] I saw that, from the schedule, the agenda, some of these were being discussed. There's prediction of life expectancy and mortality that we don't fully understand. African Americans have more strokes with the same level of blood pressure when compared to whites. And I don't know if that's because of John Henryism,

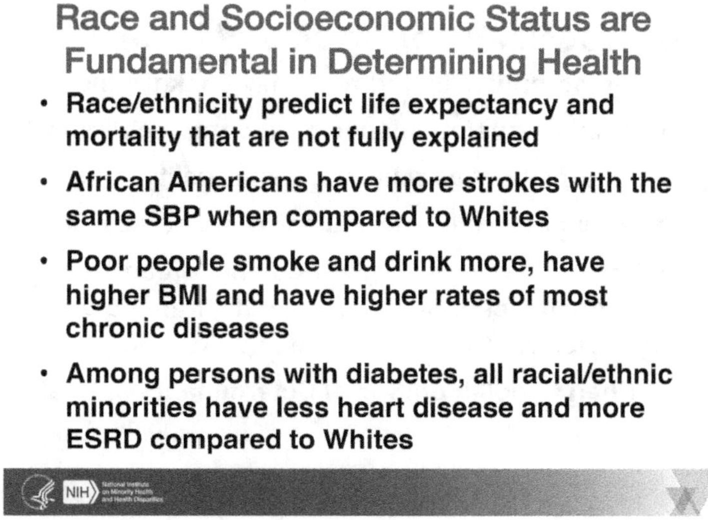

Fig. 4

racism, or socioeconomic status, but the data are very, very robust. So that, to me means that Black Americans should have their blood pressure better controlled, or at least as well controlled as whites. And we don't do that. And that's where the deficiency comes in. And poor people generally smoke more, drink more, use more substances, have higher body mass index, higher rates of most chronic diseases, not all, but most, and understanding that I think is important. Maybe the guaranteed minimum income would go some way to address that. But there are also other interventions that could be considered. And then even within the disease, such as diabetes, we see that all minority groups, which all have excess rates of diabetes, including Asians, have less heart disease. And these are data generated in part from UCSF on the Kaiser diabetes registry over a decade ago. And all have more end stage renal disease. Now, why is that? Less heart attacks, less heart failure, but more dialysis, and understanding that I think scientifically will be relevant. In this case, we also have to consider this complex playing field of social determinants that have been getting a lot of attention now at the level of the Department of Health and Human Services.

And so more will be coming from this. [Fig. 5] And this is just a brief summary of the individual determinants at top. It's not exhaustive, but you can see where I'm coming from on this. And then the structural determinants, which have been mentioned, related to all the issues of where we live in play, housing, green space, you know, to broadband internet. We really think it was that important until about 15 months ago. Economic opportunities, transportation, etc. NIMHD actually embarked on a project three years ago

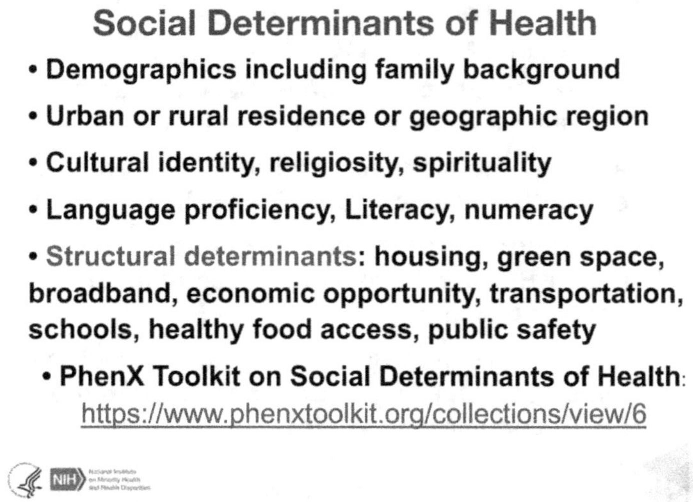
Social Determinants of Health
• Demographics including family background
• Urban or rural residence or geographic region
• Cultural identity, religiosity, spirituality
• Language proficiency, Literacy, numeracy
• Structural determinants: housing, green space, broadband, economic opportunity, transportation, schools, healthy food access, public safety
• PhenX Toolkit on Social Determinants of Health: https://www.phenxtoolkit.org/collections/view/6
NIH

Fig. 5

to develop standardized measures for the social determinants. We finished that one major component of it. A couple of UCSF faculty were part of our expert panel, Alicia Fernandez and Paula Braveman, specifically. The measures that were vetted are on the PhenX toolkit website, and the link is there in the slides. We're continuing this project and staff have developed a set of measures that we will watch to the PhenX process to try and identify in-depth measures. Most of them are focused on the structural social determinants, since the individual ones generally have mostly been covered.

On patient doctor communication issues, I'll start with just saying that in my own practice, and believe me, I'm now getting to the point where I can no longer have any credibility since it's been almost six years since I took care of patients directly. [Fig. 6] I always started my visits with patients with, who are they? and ask them about their background after the initial checkup or complaint and make sure that there wasn't any acute issue that I needed to immediately pay attention to. I wanted to know their story.

So, the way I said that to students on the wards in teaching was to get the social history first, and when you present a case to me, present the social history first after you do the one sentence on the medical scene. And I value that. I think that that connects people with patients. It's their story. Where were they born, who are they, what do they do, how far did they go in school … You get these central elements. Frequently in that interaction, I shared my own path in some ways, particularly in people who spoke Spanish, but not exclusively. And I found that most of the time, to at least have one response to

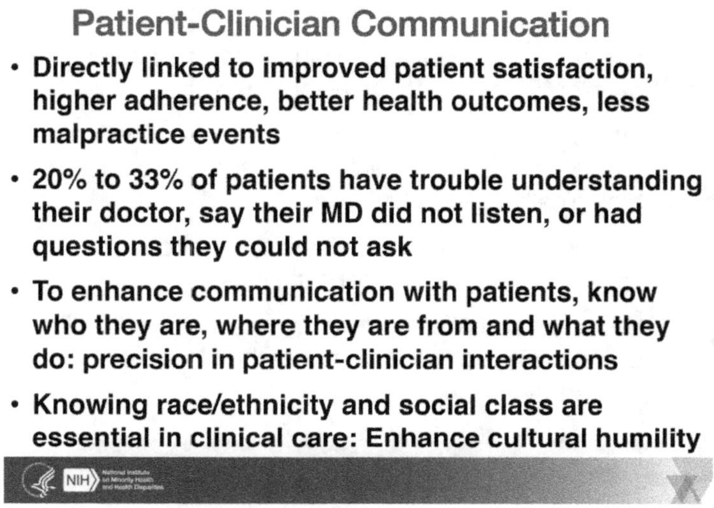

Fig. 6

Denise's question of how do you bring this up with patients, I do think that we know the power of patient clinician communication. It is an understudied area. It's directly linked to better satisfaction, better adherence, better health outcomes, and less malpractice events in one well done study.

And about a third of patients, who were disproportionately more minorities, have trouble understanding their doctor, say their MD did not listen, or have questions they couldn't not ask. And this is a when they speak the same language. These differences are magnified when you're going through

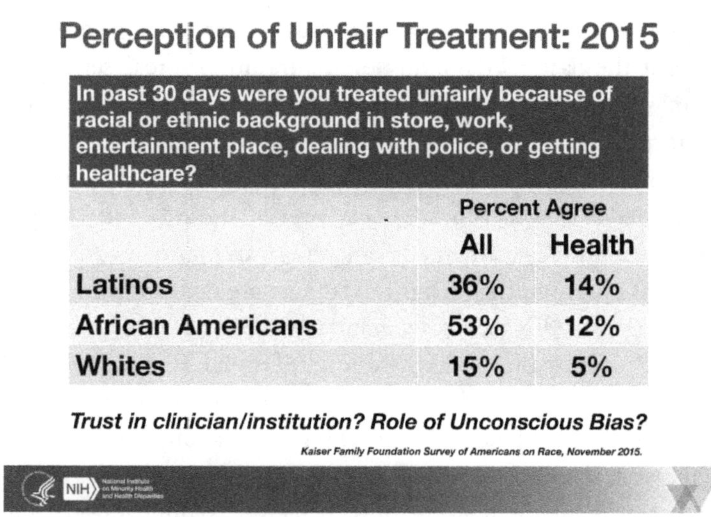

Fig. 7

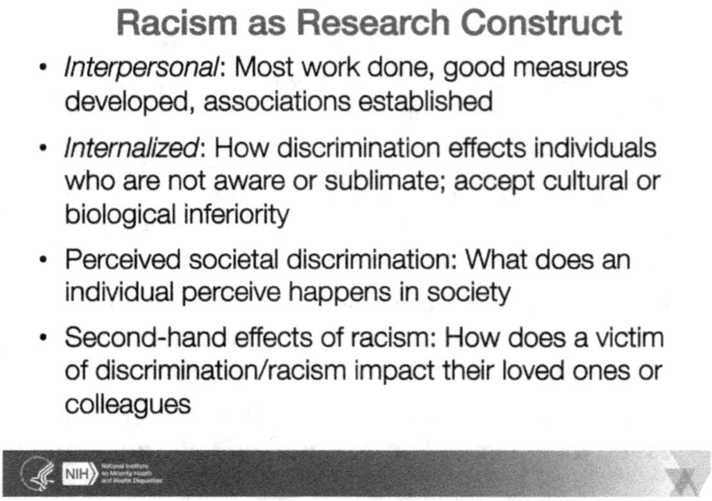

Fig. 8

an interpreter. And then to enhance communications with patients, you know, knowing who they are, I think is really essential in getting some position in patient clinician interactions. So I would argue that knowing someone's race/ethnicity in clinical care and social class, as well as their lived experience, and what did they do, what's their family like, is really a starting point for developing good rapport with patients, independent of the setting. Maybe acute issue in the emergency room doesn't really allow for that.

We've been talking about racism, and you're all familiar with this issue. This is data from six years ago, could be equally bad now or worse. [Fig. 7] When asked by a Kaiser Family Foundation national survey (and this was updated from a prior survey they had done about 15 years earlier), they asked about the past 30 days, any events in any of those settings listed there. You can see that over half of African American respondents and over a third of Latinos, all said that they had experienced this in the past 30 days. So I think I show this in almost every talk I give recently. And it's really to establish the knowledge that racism, we're not over it. It didn't end 150 years ago. It didn't end when we elected an African American president. And certainly, the issues of 2020 brought this to light. But these are not new problems. And we've been dealing with this for many, many years.

Operationalizing this as an interpersonal, internalized, and then perceived racism, which is another way of looking at some interesting studies have been done mostly with adolescents asking them about what they think is out there, not what they experience. [Fig. 8] Forty percent of 11th graders in Los Angeles, a majority of them nonwhites, perceived significant societal discrimination

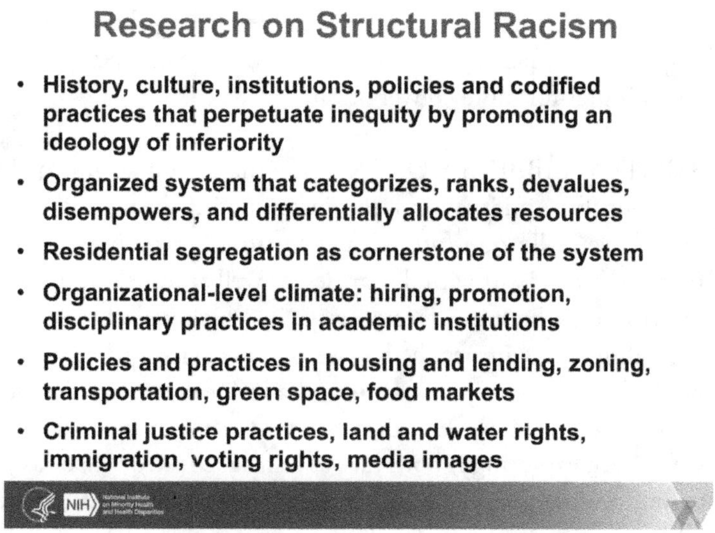

Fig. 9

against a variety of factors, not just race/ethnicity, including disability, sexual orientation, and gender. And then secondhand effects, another concept that hasn't been studied extensively. There is some literature on this, how does a victim of discrimination impact their loved ones? So those of us who've done tobacco are familiar with this concept. And clearly, it could have effects particularly on young children.

This was mentioned earlier, and I think we're really enthused that this came out. It came out with, I think almost all institutes and centers at NIH endorsed it and committed funds. So it is an RFA and we have significant amount of funds available for funding grants in fiscal 22. [Fig. 9] It will be this year that people will need to submit. This has probably been discussed in this group, but you know, recognizing that structural racism (a) exists, and (b) we should do something about it. We really need interventions. Five years ago, when I arrived at NIH, I thought, well, is this really a research construct? Can we study this? And I had been having this back-and-forth discussion about this for years with colleagues. No one really had an answer. Some people thought, well, we should propose it as an organizational theme. And perhaps in some ways, cultural competence being looked at as another concept on the opposite end of the spectrum, but regardless, I think, you know about these issues, so I won't dwell on this. And those are three bullets of topics that we outline in the RFA that really emphasizes this. We have a special issue of *Ethnicity and Diseases* being published, where we wrote a couple of commentaries and David Williams also wrote one. The papers in and of themselves are not so necessarily innovative or groundbreaking, but it's time we start to do this conversation from a science perspective, not just describing, but also really, really with emphasis on intervention. So I'll stop with that. And hopefully, we'll have a few minutes for more conversation.

KIRSTEN BIBBINS-DOMINGO: Thank you so much, Eliseo. That was really terrific. And it reminds me, just watching the ways in which you and your team have really transformed that Institute, to both expand the populations that we think about with disparities, as well as to help us to really focus on the multi layers, the multi-faceted ways in which we know that these that these large differences in health that we observe across populations really come to be, and I really love your rubric and a lot of the things that you have on your website. But you work with other ICs at the NIH and one of the themes we've been exploring is both race as a social construct that, as you say, for your definition, includes biology, but oftentimes at the NIH, by the very nature of what it does gets reduced to biology in the way other ICs might, because we tend to be reductionist in our biomedical research. That's the shorthand for it. So what do you see is your role not in not just in framing the research for us, but in your conversations will be other ICs to sort of broaden this concept of race, or at least avoid the sort of biological determinist view of race?

ELISEO PÉREZ-STABLE: So thanks for that question, Kirsten. You know, I cannot say that anyone has tried to counter my perspective. Probably the group that I've had the most conversations about at the leadership level has been genome, and it really began from day one. And we certainly don't agree 100%. I took me a while to realize that. But they're also not coming out and saying, we don't think you're this race because your ancestral markers say otherwise. NHGRI and NIMHD co-sponsored a workshop, probably, I think it was 2016. And we had a number of high-profile people come including, I think Esteban was part of that conversation. Alice Popejoy, David Hayes-Bautista, I mean, we had a number of conversations. I think the conclusion from that workshop was that self-identified race/ethnicity was the gold standard. And then we weren't questioning that. That there were biological components that were relevant to look at from a discovery science perspective, and I think in the in the pharmacogenetic realm, they clearly have had important impact on certain conditions. And then, the third conclusion I can draw from it – and we never actually published any kind of a summary (there were some documents) – was that the reality is that it's unsatisfactory to refer to self-identified race/ethnicity. People felt like, well, we need to do more, we need to do more exploration, more qualitative work, what does this really mean? And so that was one of the outcomes of that. And so I can't say that people are opposed to it. I don't see Francis Collins getting up and saying this in public, but he certainly isn't contradicting it. I don't know if that answers your question.

There are other people at NIH now. People may not have followed, besides Lindsey Criswell who came over from UCSF and the newest newbie, Shannon Zenk, who's a population scientist, Director of the National Institute of Nursing. Michael Chiang is the Director of Eye Institute. This is the first time we've ever had Eye institute interested in issues we're focusing on. He's an ophthalmologist, tech, informatics kind of person. And Deb Tucci is the otolaryngologist, an actual surgeon, is a director of the Hearing Institute. And so I think that there's sort of a new generation of leaders at NIH with perhaps a less reductionist perspective, just because, you know, Francis is actually a pretty open minded person, and he's the one who makes these decisions. And otherwise, we're not stuck in one perspective here.

KIRSTEN BIBBINS-DOMINGO: That's great. We're also, I think, many of us really happy with the RFA on structural racism that came out and really understanding that health effects of structural racism. But as you alluded to, you'd like to see more than moving just beyond description to actual intervention. And if the interventions, by definition, are highly likely to be structural in nature, how do you do that in the way that the NIH has typically thought about interventions, which tend to be for individuals, right? I mean, because it's very much in the biomedical mode.

ELISEO PÉREZ-STABLE: No, that's a good point. And I think there is a consensus that whatever is going to be done here, we're going to depend on you, our great, innovative, and bright scientists out there to come up with ideas that are out of the box. It may take other mechanisms besides this initial RFA, and we're working on that. But I think there's a clear understanding that we do need to address issues using other sectors of government and society.

So you can't get at housing, or transportation, or green space without involving other sectors of society. And I think there are generally two areas and you probably all have heard this, that may seem accessible for creating change. One is actually organizational, and relates to not just institutions, but healthcare systems. And I think that's more feasible to think about with the kind of mechanisms that we have now with this RFA in terms of R01s. And the other is thinking about healthy communities. How do we get to that? I think there's enough evidence-based interventions have what it takes to create better health in the long term. And yet, we can never really evaluate what the package would do or how we can make a difference in community. There are some examples out in society, but they're just too few. So more is to come.

This is not the only RFA. We had this RFA ready in September, and they got put on hold because of the executive order. And, I think putting it on hold had the unexpected advantage of getting every Institute on NIH to endorse it. And actually, one of the reasons that happened was because Francis asked people to do that. And although I think many would have done it anyway, having him say it in an IC directors meeting moved people to act rather than wait for, for us to ask them.

KIRSTEN BIBBINS-DOMINGO: That's terrific. Well, I know many of us really appreciate you and your leadership and the Institute continuing to push these issues forward. So thank you, Eliseo, for taking the time to join us today and for your comments. And I hope you're able to join us for the next session as well. And I think with that, we will conclude this really terrific day. And my appreciation to all of the speakers, to all of the panelists, and to all the audience members who really came through with some terrific questions. This is the first of our sets of case studies.

A week from today, we will have two case studies, one on eGFR (glomerular filtration rate) and one on polygenic risk scores. So thank you very much and I hope you all have a good rest of your day.

Introductory Remarks

Kirsten Bibbins-Domingo, PhD, MD

KIRSTEN BIBBINS-DOMINGO: Good morning. Welcome to Racism and Race: The Use of Race and Medicine and Implications for Health Equity. This is the third in our series of sessions on this topic. My name is Kirsten Bibbins-Domingo. I am the Vice Dean for Population Health and Health Equity in the UCSF School of Medicine, and I'm pleased to welcome you to today's program.

I want to begin with this number. One in one thousand. This is the lifetime risk of a Black man dying from police violence in the United States. In fact, death at the hands of the police makes police violence the leading cause of death for young men of color in the United States. It is this number and numbers like this that led the CDC to declare structural racism a public health crisis, as it did earlier this week. I want to underscore this number because it is this number and what it represents that I know many of us are bringing to our conversation today as we reflect on the ongoing events in Minneapolis, and it is this number and the number and what it represents that in fact, our patients bring into the clinical encounter, that our students bring into the classroom, and that all of us bring in to the work that we are doing, whether we are teaching, whether we are practicing, or whether we are conducting research. It's what makes the conversations that we are having both difficult and important.

I want to remind you of the shared values that we are bringing to our discussions today. We know that there will be differences of opinions as we talk about the hard work of actually applying our anti-racism principles to the work of understanding the use of race in medicine. The difference of opinion is in fact expected and welcome. We expect that all speakers and discussants are treated with respect and that, while we might have different views expressed today, that we have two common goals: advancing anti-racism in medicine and pursuing the best possible health and equitable health for all of our patients. So, this series is examining a very specific issue: how we use race in medicine and the implications for health equity. We've structured our conversation in this way.

We began on March 24th laying the foundation with historical and current perspectives. We have been engaging in a series of applied case studies and this is the second of our case studies. We'll have two during the session today. We want to really take the broader principles and see how they apply to how we generate knowledge that underlies our clinical decision making and how we teach about this body of knowledge as well. We really want to lay the groundwork in these discussions for a more intimate smaller group sets of discussions within the domains in which we practice in our in our academic medical centers: in the domains of medical care, clinical practice, and clinical and translational research. And those conversations will take place over the next several weeks.

We are dividing people up by the primary domains in which they work: education, clinical practice, and clinical and translational research. I'm really grateful to the broad group of leaders across our UC medical center campuses who've agreed to lead and help facilitate some of these discussions. This is the opportunity for the many of you who participated in our workshops up to now to really be part of smaller breakout groups to really reflect on what you've heard over these sessions as well as help us to draw out principles that might help us inform how we educate, how we practice, and how we conduct research in a better way.

I'm really grateful to many people, but I want to highlight these four. So if you joined us last week, you'll know that we started our case study with a really fabulous video that many of you commented on, and I'm really grateful to Cameron Hicks, who's one of our medical students, for developing the script for that video, as well as to Matthew Ryan, who is another of our medical students, an MD/PhD student, who developed the script for the video that you will see today in our session on polygenic risk scores. Our first video that you'll see was developed by two of our faculty, Dr. Delphine Tuot and Dr. Chi Chu. And thank you very much. These have been very popular, I think, in how people have received some of this information.

Case Study 2: Race Based Diagnosis-GFR Flash Talks

KIRSTEN BIBBINS-DOMINGO: So, for our session today, we have two case studies, which are numbers two and three in our series (the first was in Part I). And in each of these, we will begin with the video laying the groundwork for the types of details you need to know to understand the case followed by flash talks and then a moderated panel discussion. I think both of these topics, eGFR and polygenic risk scores, will be very interesting to you and will draw many of the themes we hope to delve deeper into in our discussions over the subsequent sessions.

So, let me get let us begin with our first case study of the day. I am really pleased to have two outstanding speakers, scholars, experts in this particular field and colleagues of mine. The first, Dr. Vanessa Grubbs, who is a writer. She is an Associate Professor of Medicine in the Division of Nephrology at UCSF. And Dr. Neil Powe, who's Professor of Medicine, Chief of the Medical Service at San Francisco General Hospital, and Vice Chair of the Department of Medicine at UCSF.

Following their flash talks, they will join a panel that I will moderate, and the panel will include Josh Adler, who's the Vice Dean for Clinical Affairs in the School of Medicine, Cynthia Delgado, who is Professor of Medicine and Nephrology and a Chair of a Society of Nephrology Task Force on this topic, and Dr. Steven Richmond, an alum from UCSF who is now a faculty member at Stanford University. So, with that, I think we will go into the video.

VIDEO NARRATOR: Measuring kidney function is an integral part of routine clinical practice. The most important measure of kidney function is the glomerular filtration rate, or GFR, which measures how well the kidneys filter the blood. GFR is used to guide many decisions in clinical care, including the diagnosis of chronic kidney disease, eligibility to be a kidney donor, referral to a kidney specialist, eligibility to be wait listed for a kidney transplant, and initiation of dialysis. In addition, many drugs are dosed based on GFR and some drugs may be contraindicated in patients with GFR below certain cutoffs.

Unfortunately, methods for measuring GFR directly are cumbersome and not feasible for routine clinical practice. Instead, the medical community has developed ways to obtain an estimated GFR or eGFR from routinely available lab tests. The most widely used eGFR equations use serum creatinine, a substance in the blood that is freely filtered and excreted by the kidneys. However, GFR is not the only factor that affects serum creatinine. Creatinine is steadily produced by muscle and is also influenced by diet and other unknown factors. However, because the production of creatinine is generally steady in each individual, any changes in serum creatinine are predominantly the effect of changes in GFR. Thus, creatinine serves as an indicator for GFR as long as we can account for the effects of other factors affecting serum creatinine.

Given the difficulty of measuring diet, muscle mass, as well as other unknown factors that affects serum creatinine, the scientific community developed equations that use demographic variables as surrogates for the unmeasured factors that affect creatinine. The two most common equations, called the MDRD and the CKD-EPI equations, use age, sex, and Black versus non-Black race, in addition to serum creatinine. They respectively assign a 21 and 16 higher eGFR to Black individuals compared to non-Black individuals. However, although inclusion of these demographic variables led to greater accuracy in the studies used to derive these equations, the inclusion of race is highly problematic especially since critical clinical decisions hinge on specific eGFR thresholds. eGFR equations using filtration marker alternatives to creatinine that are not epidemiologically associated with race are under investigation.

One such marker, Cystatin C is available now, though widespread adoption has been slow, assays are not widely available, and cost remains a barrier. While the scientific community looks forward to a future with accurate widely available raceless GFR markers, we're left in a predicament as to how to handle creatinine-based eGFR in the near term. How do we ensure eGFR equations are as accurate as possible for clinical decision making and research? Can we ensure that race is not being used in a way that reinforces wrong messages or produces barriers to care and health? How can we encourage productive discussions about this controversy to maintain focus on eliminating known racial disparities in health care and health outcomes?

KIRSTEN BIBBINS-DOMINGO:
Excellent. Dr. Grubbs?

If Black: The Racialization of Kidney Function

Vanessa Grubbs, MD

VANESSA GRUBBS: I'm thankful to be invited to present my perspective on this issue. I've been writing and talking about this issue publicly since 2017, but I have personally been aware of it when I started my nephrology fellowship at UCSF in 2007. [Fig. 1] Since that time, I've seen it as something problematic at best. And really, to me, it feels like we are in this predicament of having to defend the humanity of Black people as not being inherently different than every other human on the planet. So, with that, I'll just jump straight into the equations that were presented in the video.

The evidence is biased. [Fig. 2] To go into more detail in the first equation published in 1999, there were roughly 200 Black participants. The researchers put several biologic variables and self-reported Black race in the regression

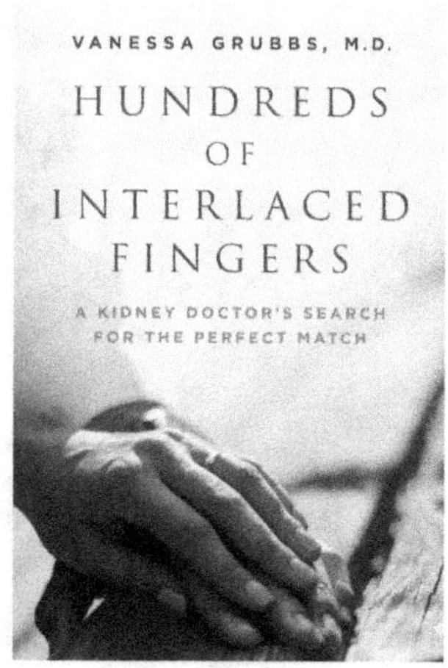

Fig. 1

HarperCollins Publishers, Amistad division
June 2017

model and kept things that had a significant p-value – a very significant p-value, I acknowledge. However, there was no *a priori* hypothesis for why kidney function might be different in Black participants.

So, after the fact, the authors asserted on average Black persons have higher muscle mass than white persons. Here are the studies that they cited. I won't go into those in any detail. I just put the basics here to show you the age of the study and how sadly small and pretty much inconsequential to proving their point about muscle mass. And then, one of the issues is that the authors did not give us an indication that the Black and white participants were otherwise the same apart from race. That data has yet to be presented or published, as far as I'm aware. But we do have this study that was based on a sub sample of the same larger study and what we can see is there was a lot higher blood pressure

THE EVIDENCE IS BIASED

- MDRD (the Modification of Diet in Renal Disease study) Equation
  Participants: Black (n=197) & White (n=1304)
  Regression model: multiple biologic variables and self-reported Black race, $p<0.001$
  No *a priori* hypothesis for why kidney function different in Black participants
- Post hoc explanation: "...on average black persons have higher muscle mass than white persons."
  - Cohn et al. 1997
    47 Black and 67 White adults
    "Blacks had higher total-body calcium and potassium than the...White population."
  - Worrall et al. 1990
    30 Black and 30 White adults
    "Racial variation in creatine kinase was independent of lean body mass."
  - Harsha et al. 1978
    99 Black and 143 White children in Louisiana
    "Black children were found to have less body fat than White children."

Levey *et al. Ann Intern Med* 1999. @thenephrologist

Fig. 2

SEPARATE AND UNEQUAL

Hebert et al. *Hypertension.* 1997.

Characteristic (%)*	*Black (n=53)*	*White (n=495)*
History of hypertension	98.1	83.8
Annual income <$25K	77.4	48.9
Hypertensive nephrosclerosis	28.3	16.0
Diabetic nephropathy	9.4	2.2

*p<0.05

Fig. 3

and a lot more diabetes in that subpopulation. [Fig 3]

There's no reason to think they would be vastly different than the larger group. These are certainly factors that might explain why the Black people in that study had a higher GFR than a given creatinine than their white counterparts. Then when we come to the CKD-EPI equation published roughly 10 years later. [Fig. 4] This is where we get that the Black othering is reified. It was a much larger patient population. It was a tiny bit more diverse, but the issue is that it started with Black versus other from the start. That's a decision. Someone decided to 'other' Black people. And as shown in the video, it reflected that if you're African American, your measured GFR was 16 higher than every other human on the planet. So, a question that I've always asked is, how Black exactly is African American?

BLACK OTHERING REIFIED

- CKD-EPI (Chronic Kidney Disease Epidemiology Collaboration) Equation
- More precise at higher GFR than MDRD
- Equation development from 8,254 participants in 10 studies
  More diverse: 5% Hispanic and Asian
  Black versus Other from start
- "if African American" × 1.16

Fig. 4

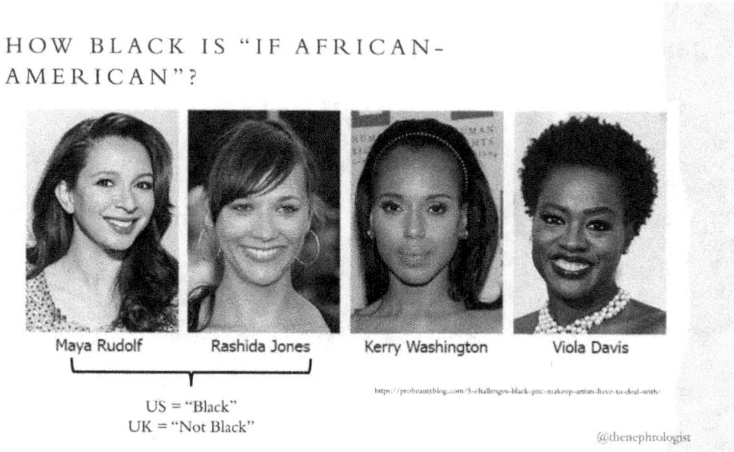

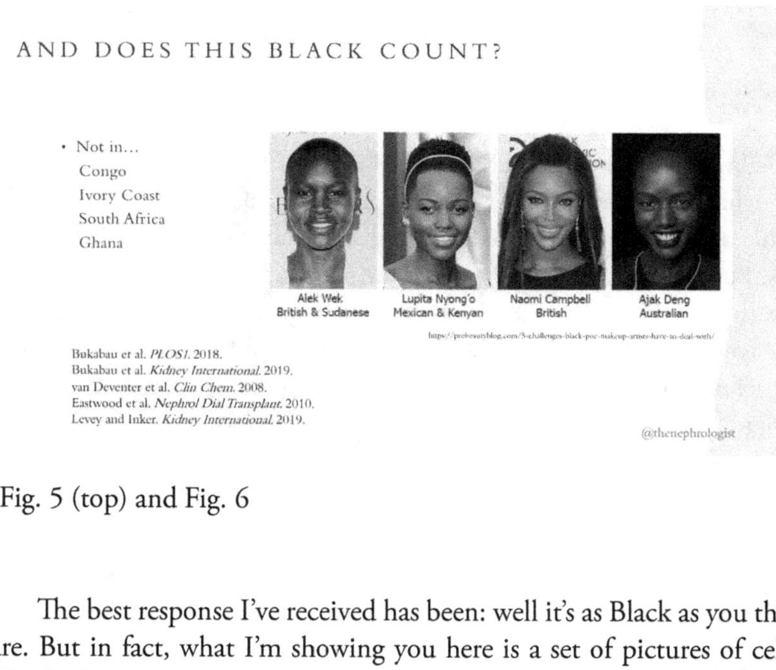

Fig. 5 (top) and Fig. 6

The best response I've received has been: well it's as Black as you think you are. But in fact, what I'm showing you here is a set of pictures of celebrities all of whom identify as Black. [Fig. 5] In the US, so because you identify as Black, yeah, you're Black. But in the UK, anyone who is biracial, such as these two celebrities, would be considered not Black. And then I've asked, well does this Black count, because these are not African Americans – all beautiful Black women celebrities as well. [Fig. 6] We've had several studies that show that this race multiplier is not valid in these African nations, and even two of the researchers from the equation development acknowledged that the race multiplier or race correction was not necessary in those countries, and perhaps the difference might be due to diet. But why none of those hypotheses could

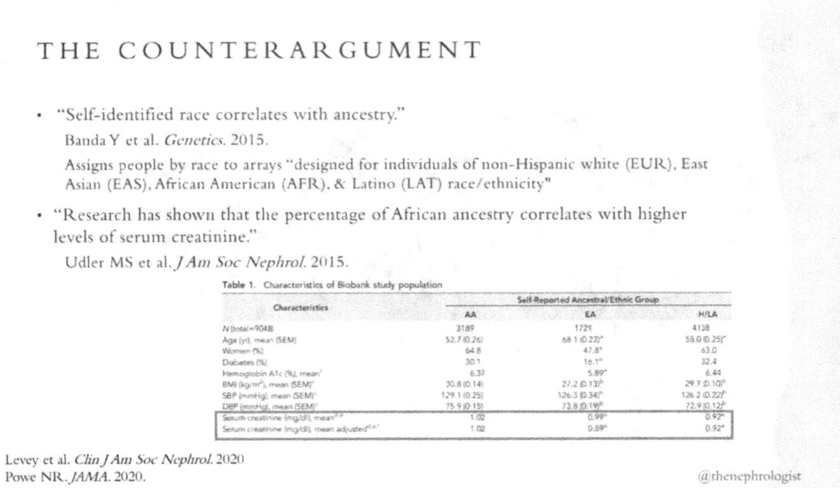

Fig. 7

be applied in this country is questionable.

So, what we have from the counter argument, at least what I've heard repeatedly and published repeatedly, is that self-identified race correlates with ancestry. But when you look into – this is the paper that's cited – everyone that's participating in this study, they're assigned to areas that are developed based on these continental stratifications. [Fig. 7] So, it should not be surprising that people defined by race, which are defined by continents, actually correlates really highly to those continents by the assigned race. So, it, to me, is kind of circular thinking.

Fig. 8

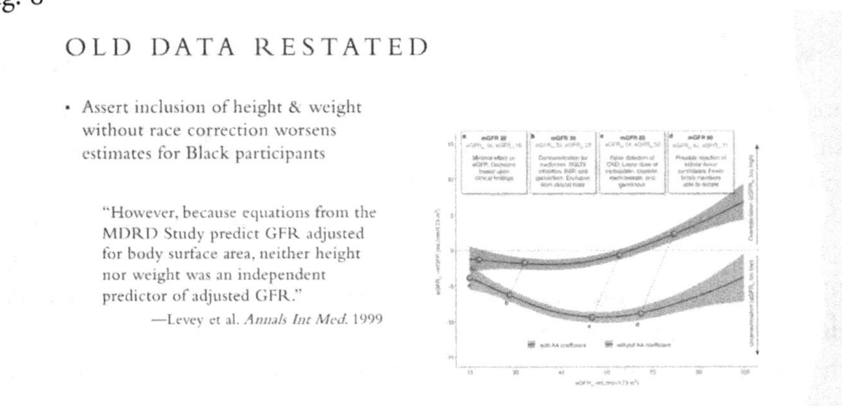

And then the other point is that the research has shown that the percentage of African ancestry correlates with higher levels of serum creatinine. Again, this is the study that is cited [Udler, et al., 2015]. Down here, we see this is the serum creatinine for the African ancestry, European, and the Hispanic/ Latino. What I want to point out here is that there is very little difference in these numbers. It's certainly not something that has much clinical meaning and when the when it's adjusted for several factors, I find it very curious that only the European mean creatinine moves as opposed to the other two. Again, I don't see that as being much of a clinical difference, and certainly not much smaller than reflected in our actual equations. And then we had this publication that basically restated the old data. [Fig. 8]

The authors present this lovely figure that shows how awful it is to not use the African American race multiplier when approaching the actual GFR here. In response to an earlier publication which suggested, *well maybe we should use other things like height and weight to replace race*, these authors asserted that when they included height and weight without the race correction, it actually worsened the estimates for the Black participants. But I'm saying this is old data restated because in the original study, the 1999 study, they talked about how because they adjusted for body surface area, neither height nor weight was an independent predictor of adjusted GFR. So, this is really just a regurgitation of things they already published, when actually, what would have been helpful would be had they presented an estimate of all the pooled data or actually showed us that the participants were otherwise the same besides race. But instead, they just double down on the same original information. I've

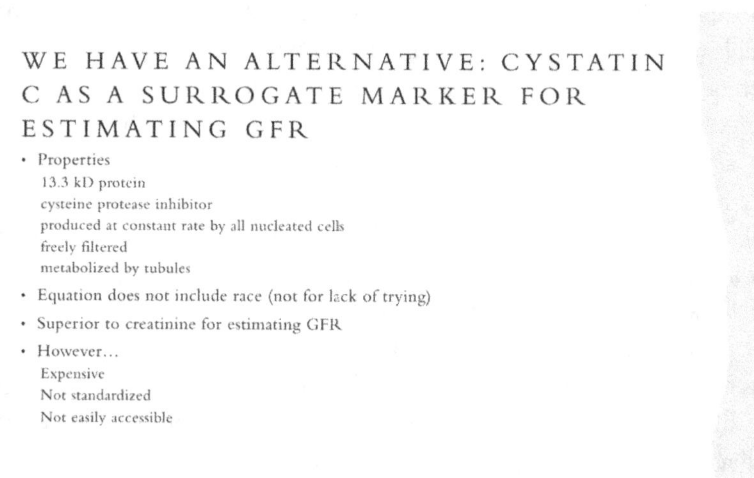

Fig. 9

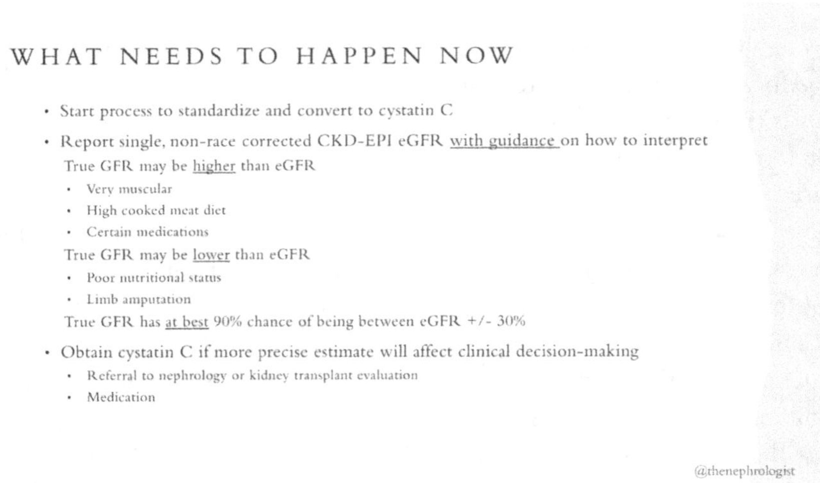

Fig. 10

heard people say, well that would take years to do.

But I think at this point, we can remind ourselves that we were able to create a vaccine in less than 10 months. So, crunching some numbers doesn't seem that impossible. However, the folks who are very much in favor of maintaining the race multiplier have all of these dramatic statements of what could happen by doing this – those medications will be denied, and people won't be able to donate a kidney, all of these various things. But I'd like to point out is that what this presumes is that the race correction is valid in the first place. So, if the race correction is not valid, and that's what we are saying, then all of these things are pretty moot. And it also assumes that by looking only through a race lens that only affects Black people, it's not considering what unintended consequences or negative effects that has on all of us. And what's particularly ridiculous about this to me is that we already have another alternative, as presented in the video. [Fig. 9] We have Cystatin C, which does not include a race correction factor. But again, I want to point out that this is not for lack of trying, because they did put it in a model. But thankfully, there just wasn't a significant p-value. And again, the researchers did not offer any hypothesis on why a protein that's produced at a constant rate by all nucleated cells might be different in Black people and only Black people.

There's been a lot of discussion about how we shouldn't just change rapidly without really thinking this through. But there is a 20-year body of literature showing that Cystatin C is superior to creatinine for estimating GFR. True,

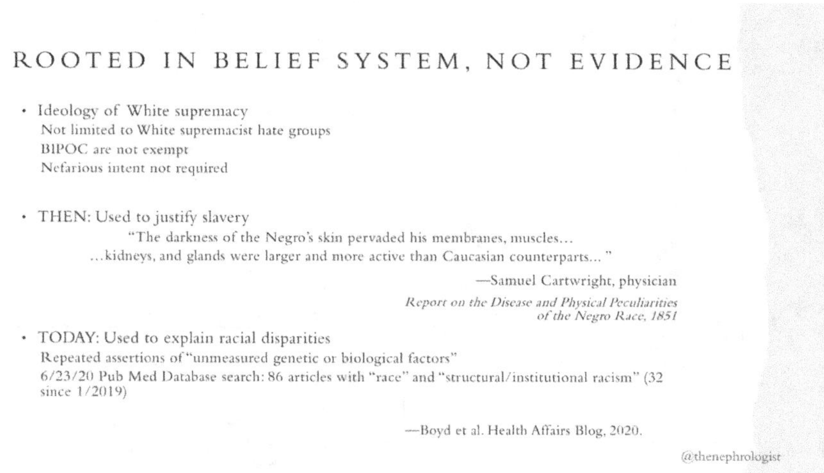

Fig. 11

it is currently expensive, not standardized, and not readily accessible. Most labs still send it out, so it takes a long time to get the result back. However, I remember in the early 2000s when we went through a very major process of standardizing creatinine as well. So, to use these things as reasons for why we should not just switch to the thing that is better and already exists is just an excuse. These are overcomeable barriers.

So, this is what I assert needs to happen now. [Fig. 10] We need to go ahead and start the process for standardizing and converting to Cystatin C. Of course, that will take some time, so in the meantime, we should report a single, non-race corrected CKD-EPI eGFR, but with some guidance on how clinicians should interpret it. Instead of just assuming that race is the only thing that they need to take into consideration, for example, the true GFR might be higher than the estimated GFR if the person is really muscular or eats a very heavy cooked meat diet. And similarly, the true GFR might be lower than the estimated if someone is very frail or has a limb amputation. And what really has been overlooked almost entirely in this national conversation over the past two and a half years is that at best, the true GFR only has a 90 chance of being the point estimate, plus or minus 30 percent. So, we're doing a lot of bickering and debate over precision that does not exist. As you recall the CKD-EPI race correction is 16%. If we need actual precision to help make important clinical decisions, that's when we can get a Cystatin C right now, when you don't need it need the result within an hour.

So, my thoughts on why this hasn't happened yet is because we and

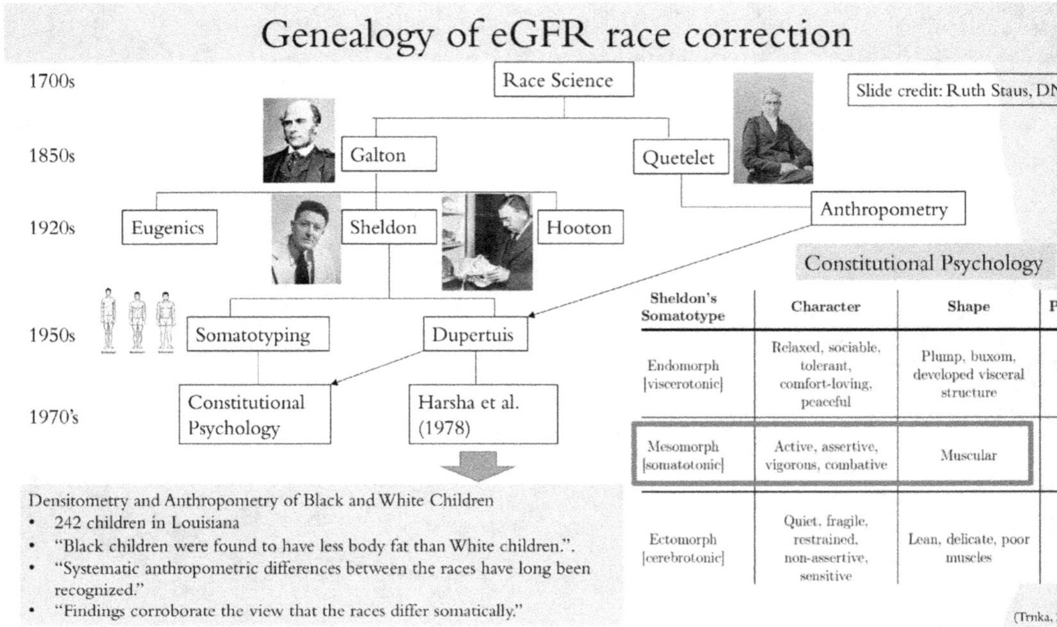

Fig. 12

biomedicine do not believe this definition of what race is that was presented in the first session by Professor Dorothy Roberts. All the social sciences have accepted that race is an invented social hierarchy to control people, but biomedical scientists, as I said, do not *en masse* accept this. And you know who else doesn't accept this? White supremacists.

So, to me, this is what it gets down to – what is really going on – all of this conversation is not about evidence. It's really about a belief system that is rooted in an ideology of white supremacy. And not to confuse it with white supremacist hate groups – this is not what I'm talking about. Contrary to what seems to be repeatedly suggested, just because someone is of color doesn't mean they're not capable of upholding the same ideology. And intent does not matter. Impact is what has the consequences. So, in the past, we've used it to justify slavery. [Fig. 11] Also, as Professor Roberts mentioned, this physician Samuel Cartwright, reporting on the peculiarities of the negro race, made lots of statements without any data, and also specifically mentioned the kidneys, and all of these things made them better, make the negro race better equipped for being enslaved. And today we're doing just a different iteration, where we're trying to use it to explain racial disparities.

Some of our colleagues recently published in the *Health Affairs* blog

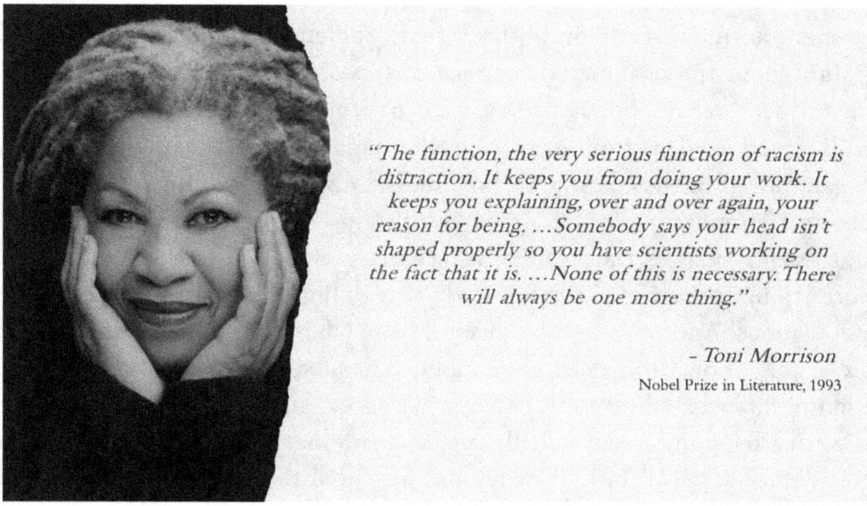
"The function, the very serious function of racism is distraction. It keeps you from doing your work. It keeps you explaining, over and over again, your reason for being. ...Somebody says your head isn't shaped properly so you have scientists working on the fact that it is. ...None of this is necessary. There will always be one more thing."
- Toni Morrison
Nobel Prize in Literature, 1993

what we've all seen. Almost every paper has repeated assertions that there's unmeasured genetic or biological factors that might really explain why there are these disparities. Within that paper, they also did a PubMed database search. In the history, there were only 86 articles that actually mentioned race and structural or institutional racism. And 32 of those studies have been since the pandemic.

So, what I want to show you is how none of this stuff came out of the blue. This is a slide that I've adapted a tiny bit and borrowed from Ruth Staus that shows the real genealogy of how we got to the GFR race correction. [Fig. 12] It started with this race science – we get the eugenics, anthropometry, and then all of this somatotyping about who the Black man is. And this is the mesomorph and with character traits and the shape of their body is being very muscular. All of this comes down into the 1970s when we get this article. I hope you recognize the lead author, because this is one of the studies that Levy and colleagues cited to justify why the Black race correction was needed.

And again, this was a very small study of Black children, and within the paper they made statements that these differences have long been recognized and corroborate the view that the races differ somatically. So here we are in this place of maintaining the *status quo*. And something that was really profound to me from the first session in this series is something that David Jones said, pointing out the asymmetry that race correction was inserted without really any evident debate, but somehow, we can't stop it without extensive debate. This is very evident from our ASN/NKF task force, the two largest kidney organizations in the country (at least for the ASN, the world). It was formed about 10 months ago and urged institutions to make no changes. They did recently release a report that agrees that we should not have race-based correction, but we need further study and calling for data for more diverse populations. And of course, by diverse, we're talking about racial diversity, so we're going down this exact same rabbit hole of suggesting that there's some kind of biological differences between the races. Instead, why can't we define diversity by things that actually affect creatinine production or clearance, like diet, like if you have diabetes and how well that diabetes is controlled. We really have an obsession with this biological race that I think needs to be addressed. I'll leave you with this quote from the late Toni Morrison of exactly what is happening here. [Fig. 13] Thank you.

KIRSTEN BIBBINS-DOMINGO: Thank you very much. Dr. Powe?

Race and Kidney Function

Neil Powe, MD

NEIL POWE: Okay. Good morning, everyone. I am happy to be here. Let me start with something personal. [Fig. 1] This picture in the lower left-hand corner is from a 1972 keepsake of my late father. He was born in the delta in Mound Bayou, Mississippi, came to Philadelphia after growing up in Louisiana, and got the very best job he could at that time as an administrative officer in the Philadelphia health department. On Saturdays, he often took me to work when he went to open the doors at one of the health centers he oversaw. There, I met a physician named Dr. John Simmons, a Black physician who came to the health center on weekends to provide care to indigent patients. I watched the smile on patients when they saw a Black doctor, but what more amazed me about Dr. Simmons was his command of biology and medicine and how he used the best science to deliver care. His patients trusted his care. Not surprising that when as a junior faculty work member working in outcomes research and kidney disease, I took note of the hyper disparities in kidney disease and made it part of my scholarship, trying to understand why

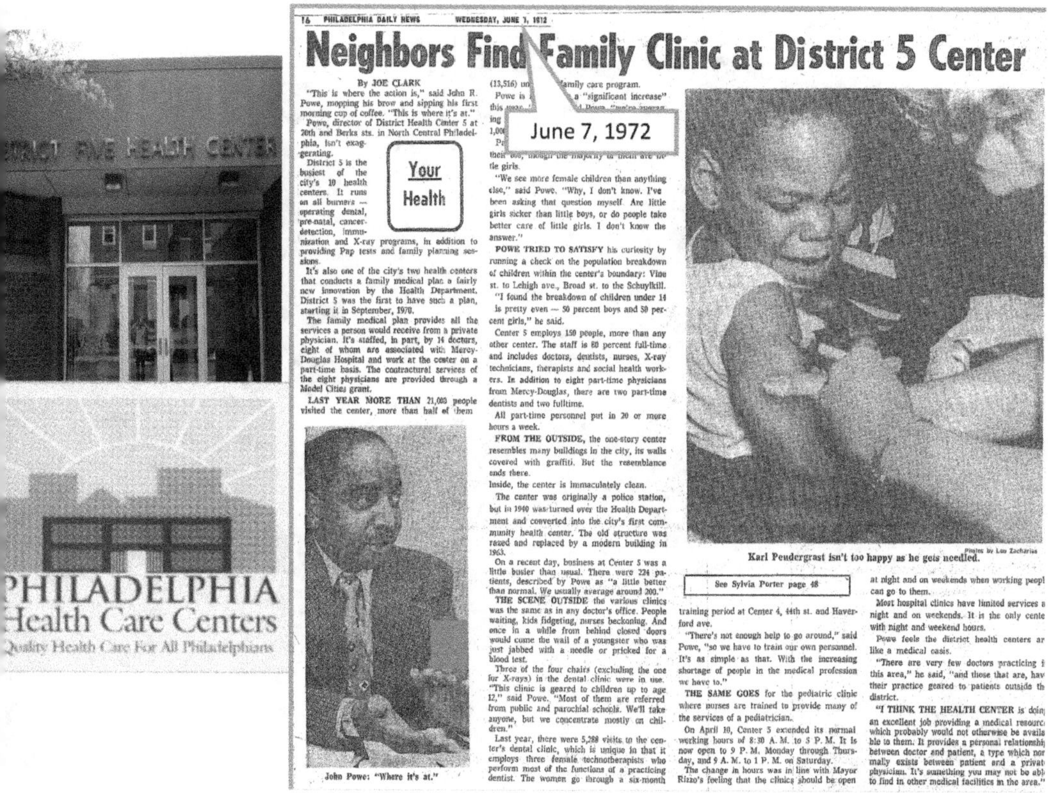

16 PHILADELPHIA DAILY NEWS WEDNESDAY, JUNE 7, 1972

Neighbors Find Family Clinic at District 5 Center

By JOE CLARK

"This is where the action is," said John R. Powe, mopping his brow and sipping his first morning cup of coffee. "This is where it's at."

Powe, director of District Health Center 5 at 20th and Berks sts. in North Central Philadelphia, isn't exaggerating.

District 5 is the busiest of the city's 10 health centers. It runs on all burners — operating dental, pre-natal, cancer-detection, immunization and X-ray programs, in addition to providing Pap tests and family planning sessions.

It's also one of the city's two health centers that conducts a family medical plan a fairly new innovation by the Health Department. District 5 was the first to have such a plan, starting it in September, 1970.

The family medical plan provides all the services a person would receive from a private physician. It's staffed, in part, by 14 doctors, eight of whom are associated with Mercy-Douglas Hospital and work at the center on a part-time basis. The contractural services of the eight physicians are provided through a Model Cities grant.

LAST YEAR MORE THAN 21,083 people visited the center, more than half of them (13,516) un[...] family care program.

Powe is [...] a "significant increase" this [...]

[...] the girls.

"We see more female children than anything else," said Powe. "Why, I don't know. I've been asking that question myself. Are little girls sicker than little boys, or do people take better care of little girls. I don't know the answer."

POWE TRIED TO SATISFY his curiosity by running a check on the population breakdown of children within the center's boundary: Vine st. to Lehigh ave., Broad st. to the Schuylkill.

"I found the breakdown of children under 14 is pretty even — 50 percent boys and 50 percent girls," he said.

Center 5 employs 150 people, more than any other center. The staff is 80 percent full-time and includes doctors, dentists, nurses, X-ray technicians, therapists and social health workers. In addition to eight part-time physicians from Mercy-Douglas, there are two part-time dentists and two fulltime.

All part-time personnel put in 20 or more hours a week.

FROM THE OUTSIDE, the one-story center resembles many buildings in the city, its walls covered with graffiti. But the resemblance ends there.

Inside, the center is immaculately clean.

The center was originally a police station, but in 1940 was turned over the Health Department and converted into the city's first community health center. The old structure was razed and replaced by a modern building in 1963.

On a recent day, business at Center 5 was a little busier than usual. There were 224 patients, described by Powe as "a little better than normal. We usually average around 200."

THE SCENE OUTSIDE the various clinics was the same as in any doctor's office. People waiting, kids fidgeting, nurses beckoning. And once in a while from behind closed doors would come the wail of a youngster who was just jabbed with a needle or pricked for a blood test.

Three of the four chairs (excluding the one for X-rays) in the dental clinic were in use. "This clinic is geared to children up to age 12," said Powe. "Most of them are referred from public and parochial schools. We'll take anyone, but we concentrate mostly on children."

Last year, there were 5,288 visits to the center's dental clinic, which is unique in that it employs three female technotherapists who perform most of the functions of a practicing dentist. The women go through a six-month training period at Center 4, 44th st. and Haverford ave.

"There's not enough help to go around," said Powe, "so we have to train our own personnel. It's as simple as that. With the increasing shortage of people in the medical profession we have to."

THE SAME GOES for the pediatric clinic where nurses are trained to provide many of the services of a pediatrician.

On April 10, Center 5 extended its normal working hours of 8:30 A. M. to 5 P. M. It is now open to 9 P. M. Monday through Thursday, and 9 A. M. to 1 P. M. on Saturday.

The change in hours was in line with Mayor Rizzo's feeling that the clinics should be open at night and on weekends when working people can go to them.

Most hospital clinics have limited services at night and on weekends. It is the only center with night and weekend hours.

Powe feels the district health centers are like a medical oasis.

"There are very few doctors practicing in this area," he said, "and those that are, have their practice geared to patients outside the district.

"I THINK THE HEALTH CENTER is doing an excellent job providing a medical resource which probably would not otherwise be available to them. It provides a personal relationship between doctor and patient, a type which normally exists between patient and a private physician. It's something you may not be able to find in other medical facilities in the area."

See Sylvia Porter page 48

John Powe: "Where it's at."

Photos by Lou Zacharias

Karl Pendergrast isn't too happy as he gets needled.

Fig. 1

disparities exist and how to address them. [Fig. 2] And here's a sample of the work done by me and numerous talented mentees, often under-represented minorities and women.

So, I was surprised to hear the chatter last year. Here's what I heard:

race was introduced in measurement of kidney function to be racist;

disparities in specialist referral and waitlisting were caused by putting race in equations to estimate GFR;

Black persons do not have different creatinine levels than whites;

investigators assign race in studies that developed the equations; and

normalizing Black persons to the white person standard will solve the problem.

Well, I'd like the posit that all of these are myths and I'm going to show you why I believe they are myths. That chatter drove me to write this piece last August [*JAMA* 324 (2020)]. [Fig. 3] I said that Black kidney function matters

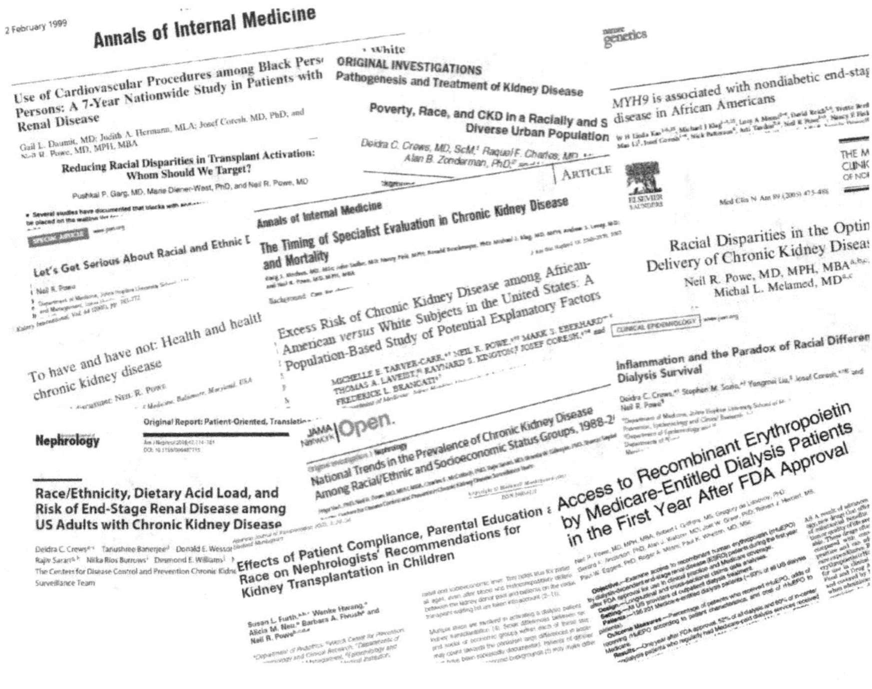

2 February 1999
Annals of Internal Medicine
Use of Cardiovascular Procedures among Black Persons: A 7-Year Nationwide Study in Patients with Renal Disease
Reducing Racial Disparities in Transplant Activation: Whom Should We Target?
ORIGINAL INVESTIGATIONS
Pathogenesis and Treatment of Kidney Disease
Poverty, Race, and CKD in a Racially and S Diverse Urban Population
ARTICLE
MYH9 is associated with nondiabetic end-stag disease in African Americans
Let's Get Serious About Racial and Ethnic I
Annals of Internal Medicine
The Timing of Specialist Evaluation in Chronic Kidney Disease and Mortality
Racial Disparities in the Optin Delivery of Chronic Kidney Diseas
Neil R. Powe, MD, MPH, MBA
Michal L. Melamed, MD
Excess Risk of Chronic Kidney Disease among African-American versus White Subjects in the United States: A Population-Based Study of Potential Explanatory Factors
To have and have not: Health and healtl chronic kidney disease
Inflammation and the Paradox of Racial Differen Dialysis Survival
Nephrology
JAMA Network Open.
National Trends in the Prevalence of Chronic Kidney Disease Among Racial/Ethnic and Socioeconomic Status Groups, 1988-2
Access to Recombinant Erythropoietin by Medicare-Entitled Dialysis Patients in the First Year After FDA Approval
Race/Ethnicity, Dietary Acid Load, and Risk of End-Stage Renal Disease among US Adults with Chronic Kidney Disease
Effects of Patient Compliance, Parental Education and Race on Nephrologists' Recommendations for Kidney Transplantation in Children

Fig. 2

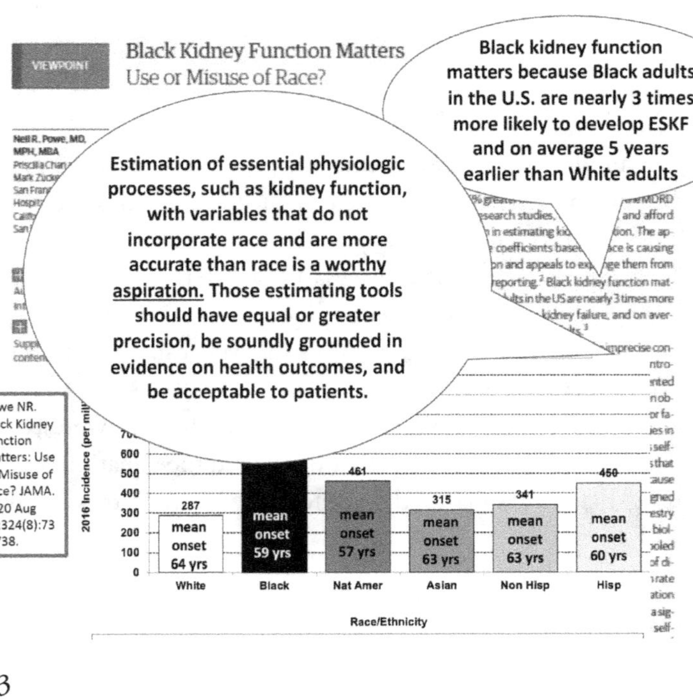

VIEWPOINT
Black Kidney Function Matters
Use or Misuse of Race?
Neil R. Powe, MD, MPH, MBA
Black kidney function matters because Black adults in the U.S. are nearly 3 times more likely to develop ESKF and on average 5 years earlier than White adults
Estimation of essential physiologic processes, such as kidney function, with variables that do not incorporate race and are more accurate than race is a worthy aspiration. Those estimating tools should have equal or greater precision, be soundly grounded in evidence on health outcomes, and be acceptable to patients.
Powe NR. Black Kidney Function Matters: Use or Misuse of Race? JAMA. 2020 Aug 25;324(8):737-738.
2016 Incidence (per mil
287
mean onset 64 yrs
mean onset 59 yrs
461
mean onset 57 yrs
315
mean onset 63 yrs
341
mean onset 63 yrs
450
mean onset 60 yrs
White
Black
Nat Amer
Asian
Non Hisp
Hisp
Race/Ethnicity

Fig. 3

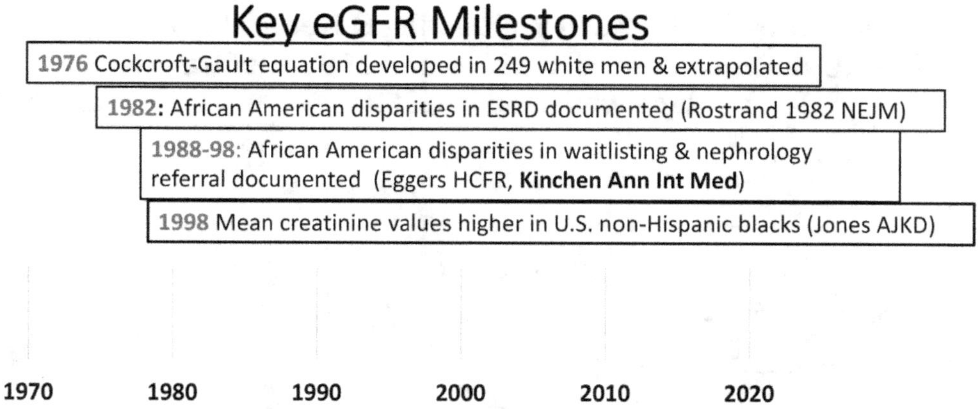

Fig. 4

because Black adults in the US are nearly three times more likely to develop end-stage kidney failure and on average five years earlier than white adults. I also said this: estimation of essential physiologic processes such as kidney function with variables that do not incorporate race and are more accurate than race is a worthy aspiration. Those estimating tools should have equal or greater precision, be soundly grounded in evidence on outcomes, and most importantly, be acceptable to patients.

So let me give you my history of eGFR measurement. [Fig. 4] In 1976, the Cockcroft-Gault equation for creatinine clearance was developed in 249 white men and extrapolated for over two decades to both women and all ethnic minorities. In 1982, there was a seminal publication in the *New England Journal* that documented the African American disparities in ESRD that I just mentioned. In 1988 through 1998, African American disparities in waitlisting and nephrology referral were well documented for over a decade by Paul Eggers and by Craig Kinchen, an African American fellow of mine who wrote this article in the *Annals of Internal Medicine.*

In 1998, there was a published report by Camille Jones that showed that mean creatinine values were higher in US non-Hispanic Blacks. Here's the data from that study. This is published in the *American Journal Kidney Diseases.* Camille jones was working at the NIH, and these are her NIH colleagues, but also notice her sister Camara Jones, who has written about the allegories of racism, was a co-author on this article. And you can see that both Black men and Black women have higher serum creatinines than the US population from nationally represented data. And this is what they said in the conclusion: [Fig. 5] "In the absence of information on GFR or lean body mass, it is not

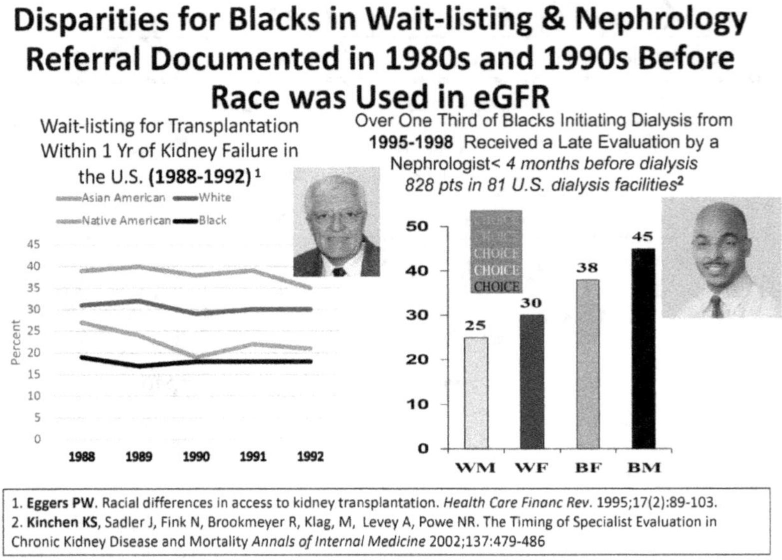
Disparities for Blacks in Wait-listing & Nephrology Referral Documented in 1980s and 1990s Before Race was Used in eGFR
Wait-listing for Transplantation Within 1 Yr of Kidney Failure in the U.S. (1988-1992) 1
Asian American
White
Native American
Black
Percent
1988
1989
1990
1991
1992
Over One Third of Blacks Initiating Dialysis from 1995-1998 Received a Late Evaluation by a Nephrologist< 4 months before dialysis
828 pts in 81 U.S. dialysis facilities2
CHOICE
25
30
38
45
WM
WF
BF
BM
1. Eggers PW. Racial differences in access to kidney transplantation. Health Care Financ Rev. 1995;17(2):89-103.
2. Kinchen KS, Sadler J, Fink N, Brookmeyer R, Klag, M, Levey A, Powe NR. The Timing of Specialist Evaluation in Chronic Kidney Disease and Mortality Annals of Internal Medicine 2002;137:479-486

Fig. 5

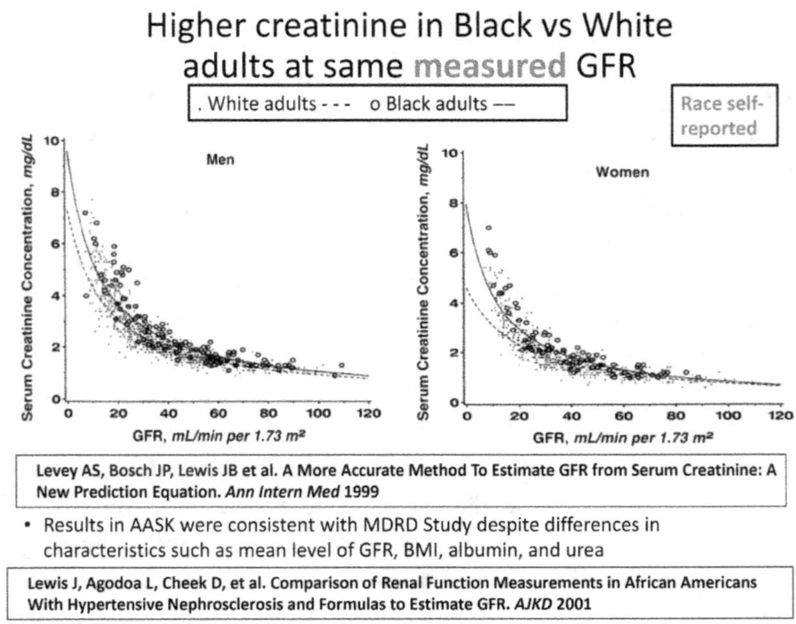
Higher creatinine in Black vs White adults at same measured GFR
. White adults - - - o Black adults —
Race self-reported
Men
Women
Serum Creatinine Concentration, mg/dL
GFR, mL/min per 1.73 m²
Levey AS, Bosch JP, Lewis JB et al. A More Accurate Method To Estimate GFR from Serum Creatinine: A New Prediction Equation. Ann Intern Med 1999
• Results in AASK were consistent with MDRD Study despite differences in characteristics such as mean level of GFR, BMI, albumin, and urea
Lewis J, Agodoa L, Cheek D, et al. Comparison of Renal Function Measurements in African Americans With Hypertensive Nephrosclerosis and Formulas to Estimate GFR. AJKD 2001

Fig. 6

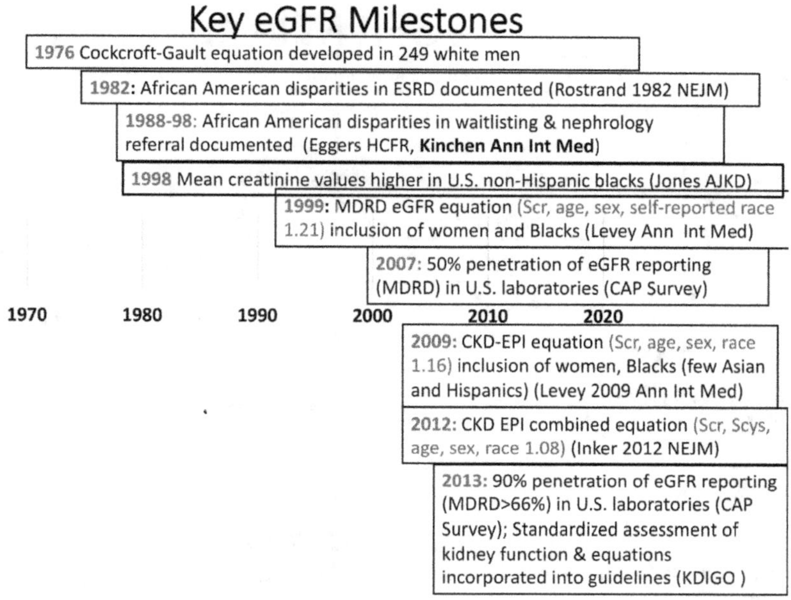

Fig. 7

clear to what extent the variability by sex, ethnicity, and age reflects normal physiologic differences rather than the presence of kidney disease. Until this information is known, the use of a single cut point to define elevated serum creatinines may be misleading." And so, a year later, as Dr. Grubbs said, the MDRD equation was published that included serum creatinine, age, sex, and self-reported race with a race modifier for African Americans and they included women and Blacks for the first time in 20 years. A similar situation happened to Framingham if you know what has happened in heart disease. And this is what they did – they had a gold standard now of measured GFR, and what they showed is that there were higher creatinine levels in Black versus white adults at the same measured GFR. [Fig. 6] So, GFR reporting was then encouraged. But you can see it took eight years to 2007 that there was 50% penetration of eGFR reporting in US laboratories. [Fig. 7]

In 2009, the CKD-EPI equation was developed. That actually included an even more diverse population of Asians and Hispanics. Unfortunately, the Asians and Hispanics were a very small minority of the population, and although there was the signal that's published in *Kidney International* by a paper by Inker, they decided not to include that coefficient for Asians because of the sample size. And then in 2012, they modified the equation to have the CKD-EPI equation that includes both serum creatinine and serum cystatin, which is

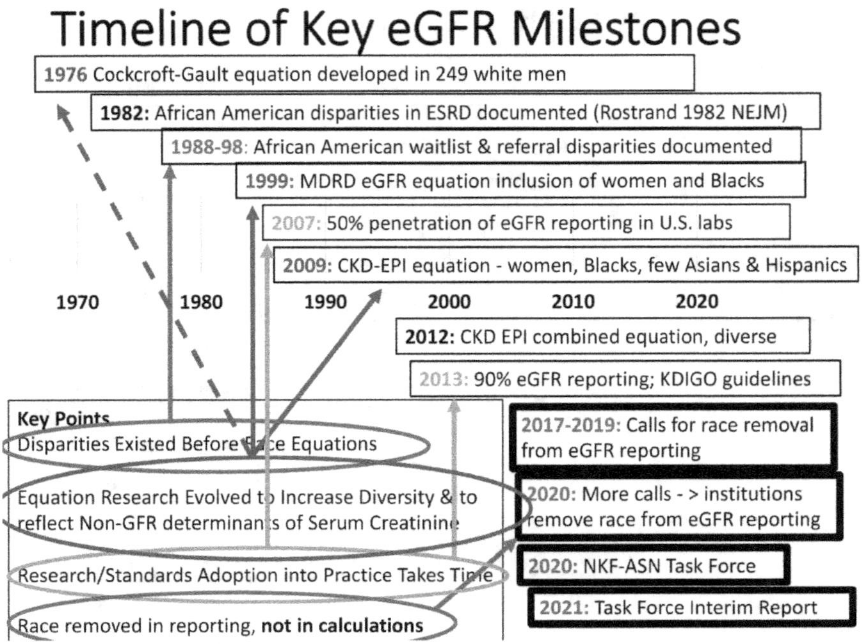

Fig. 8

even more accurate than either cystatin equations or creatinine equations. And you see it still has a mild race modifier. It took till 2013, 14 years, for there to be 90% penetration of eGFR reporting in US laboratories. And in 2013, the standardized assessment of kidney function equations was incorporated into clinical practice guidelines. In 2017-2019 there were calls for removal of race from eGFR reporting and more calls last year and institutions beginning to do that.

As Dr. Grubbs said, in 2020 the NKF back in August and the ASN, established the task force to look into this because of the importance of it. And the task force interim report was released last Friday, and I'll discuss that in a minute. But here's the key point: disparities existed before the race equations were put into existence. [Fig. 8] Equation research evolved to increase diversity and to reflect the non-GFR determinants of serum creatinine. Another point, very important, is that research standards and adoption into practice takes time. And another thing is that race has been removed in reporting the way that people have done things, but not in the calculations. So here is the interim report of the NFK-ASN task force that was published online in April of 2020. [Fig. 9] We can put that in the link for those of you who want to look at this. The task force sought a wide range of evidence and views with diverse

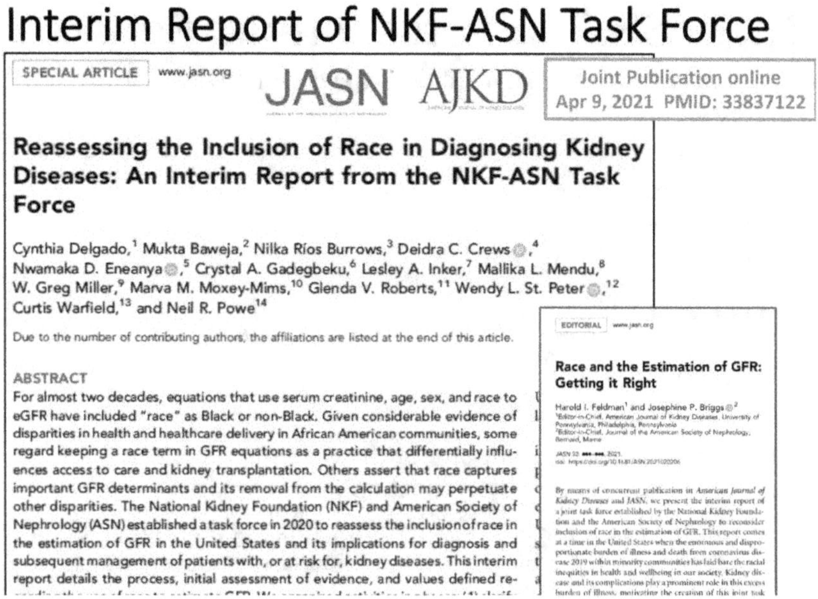

Fig. 9

representation: 16 sessions, 90 people from 19 US states and seven countries testified and the task force developed statements of evidence and value. If you look at the report, there are almost 100 references in there to information and evidence from the literature. These will form a cornerstone in forging a path forward. [Fig. 10] The task force also came up with an inventory of 26 different approaches that could be used to estimate and report kidney function, some with race some without race, and most importantly, a set of attributes to be considered in making a final recommendation among those alternative approaches.

So let me go through some of these approaches that I talked about in my article last August. [Fig. 11] The first approach, which seems to be the most common approach for those who want to eliminate race, is to take what I call the dominant race standard – discards the race coefficient and reports the non-Black coefficient. I believe it's discriminatory because it ignores data on Black persons from studies included in equation derivation, and it's less accurate for Black persons but not for white persons. You can see some of the institutions that have done it and there are potential clinical and health consequences that Dr. Grubbs pointed out. People point to the benefit that it will increase referral to specialists and access to the transplant waiting list, but there are a number

NKF-ASN Task Force Interim Report

- Sought wide range of evidence & views with diverse representation
  - **16 sessions: 90 people from 19 U.S. states and 7 countries**
- **Statements of Evidence and Value n=30: cornerstone in forging a path forward**
  - Equity and disparities
  - Race and racism
  - GFR measurement, estimation, and equation performance
  - Laboratory standardization
  - Patient perspectives
- **Inventory of 26 different approaches** to estimating and reporting estimated kidney function.
- **Attributes to be considered** in making final recommendation among alternative approaches to estimation of kidney function.

Fig. 10

Approaches to Mitigate Use of Race in eGFR Measurement or Reporting

Approach	Advantages or Challenges
Dominant ("Normalizing") Race Standard: Discard race coefficient from equations & report "non-Black" estimate B&W, MGH, VUMC, UW	Is discriminatory because it ignores data on Black persons from studies included in equation derivation. Less accurate for Black persons but not White persons.

Potential Clinical & Health Consequences

Increase in persons with CKD and more severe stages

Past underdiagnosis, or with change, overdiagnosis?

Benefit — **Balance sheet?** — **Harm**

Benefit:

↑**Referral to specialists**

↑**Access to transplant waitlist**

↑Access to Medicare services:

↑nutrition therapy

↑CKD education

↑More aggressive CKD mgmt

Powe NR. Black Kidney Function Matters: Use or Misuse of Race? JAMA. 2020 Aug 25;324(8):737-738.

Harm:

↓Living kidney donation

↓Drug use or dosing: **metformin,** SGLT2 Inh, pain meds (analgesics, opioids), ACE inhibitors, antibiotics, chemotherapy (e.g. carboplatin)

↓Contrasted Imaging procedures

↓Access to clinical trials

↑Anxiety (labeling)

Fig. 11

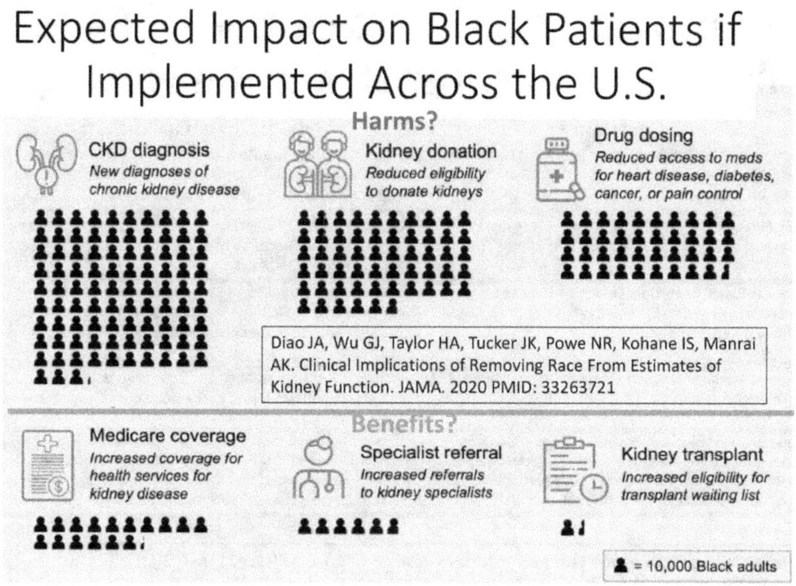

Fig. 12

of harms: decreasing live kidney donation, curtailing the use or dosing of important medications like metformin (for which disparities have already been demonstrated, and pain control in African Americans has been demonstrated to be sub-optimal), as well as decreased contrast image procedures, could decrease access to clinical trials by patients being excluded, and anxiety and labeling, and perhaps prevent people from getting life insurance. So, the stakes are high. And here's the irony of this – the expected impact on Black patients in the United States (for those things that I showed you – the harms on the right-hand side of that previous slide), the number of people affected are far greater than those affected by specialist referral and kidney transplant. [Fig. 12] So, we could hurt a lot of African Americans.

The second approach that gets used, I call racial phenotyping, and this was something that was done unfortunately at ZSFGH when advocates wanted to rapidly change how GFR was reported. [Fig. 13] So, you substitute "low muscle mass" and "high muscle mass" for non-Black and Black. Well, I think that's racist because it assumes race is a proxy for muscle mass and it stereotypes all Blacks as having muscle mass by attaching that to their coefficient, and it's less accurate for Blacks.

The third way is what I call raceless range reporting. This was first adopted

Approaches to Mitigate Use of Race in eGFR Measurement or Reporting

Approach	Advantages or Challenges
Dominant ("Normalizing") Race Standard: Discard race coefficient from equations & report "non-Black" estimate B&W, VUMC, UW	Is discriminatory because it ignores data on Black persons from studies included in equation derivation. Less accurate for Black persons but not White persons.
Racial Phenotyping: Substitute "low muscle mass" and "high muscle mass' for "non Black" and "Black" ZSFG	Assumes race is a proxy for muscle mass, thereby stereotyping all Blacks as having high muscle mass. Likely less accurate for Blacks.
Raceless Range Reporting: Report two values currently generated by the CKD Epi equation, but not openly tag them with race descriptors BIDMC, UCSF, NYU, UCI	Recognizes participation of Blacks in derivation studies and imprecision of eGFR. Leaves clinical correlation, nephrology consultation, and shared decision-making to ordering physicians.
Raceless Markers: Use non-creatinine clearance markers (e.g cystatin)	Possibly less standardization and less accurate than eGFR with creatinine. Not tested in sick populations. Higher cost.
Blended Race Standard: Develop new equation from CKD-EPI data using weighted average of ethnicity coefficients (e.g. 32% of CKD Epi Black participants, 13% in U.S. or % of Blacks at a health care institution)	Requires agreement on appropriate weights. Raises question whether same should be done for all race/ethnic groups. Likely less accurate for both Black and non Black persons but may be equitable and acceptable.

Powe NR. Black Kidney Function Matters: Use or Misuse of Race. JAMA 2020; 324(8): 737-738. PMID: 32761164.

Fig. 13

Summary

- Elimination of race for eGFR is a worthy aspiration, but consequences are far reaching
- Making changes is not a trivial task – seek "correct diagnosis" not "under or over diagnosis"
  → **Avoid doing more harm than good (primum non nocere)**
- Use of many approaches across the U.S. will make it difficult to understand GFR change when a patient receives care in different settings or institutions
- Some approaches promulgated to remove race institutionalize discrimination, or may be racist
- Solution should be consistent, durable, evidence-based and devised with input of clinicians, system leaders, social scientists and **patients**

Fig. 14

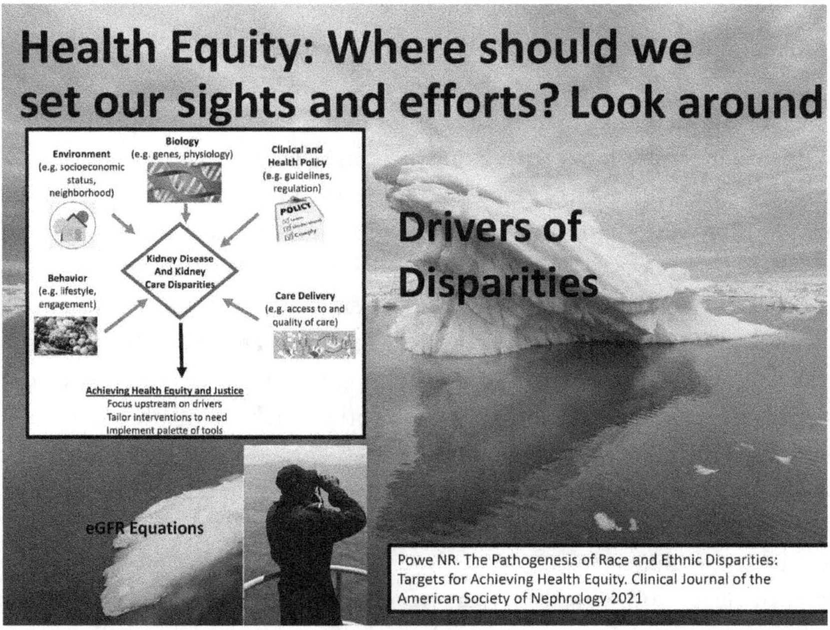

Fig. 15

by the Beth Israel Deaconess Medical Center in 2017 and has been adopted at UCSF Health, UC Irvine and NYU. And you report two values currently generated by the CKDF equation, but you don't openly tag them with race descriptors. So, this recognizes the participation in Blacks in derivation studies and it also recognizes that eGFR, as Dr. Grubbs said, is imprecise, and it leaves clinical correlation, nephrology consultation, and shared decision making to ordering physicians. And then there's the raceless marker approach, the use of non-creatinine markers, and Cystatin C is just one of them. Dr. Grubbs pointed out some of the problems, so I won't get go into those. But one additional problem is we know far less about cystatin and most of the studies have been done in ambulatory populations, not tested in sick populations, and we know that Cystatin C is an acute phase reactant and may not perform well in sicker patients.

And last, there's what I call the blended race standard, and what this is, you could develop a new equation that would weight the participants in the study and come up with a raceless equation that could be applied to everyone. But, if you just use Black and white, it raises the question whether it should be done for all races. And here's the irony of this – it's less likely to be accurate for both Black and non-Black patients, but it may be equitable and acceptable.

And that could have been done some 20 years ago, but that's what you would have had.

So, in summary, elimination of race for eGFR is a worthy aspiration, but the consequences are far reaching and making changes is not a trivial task. [Fig. 14] We seek the correct diagnosis, not under or over diagnosis. We want to avoid doing more harm than good when we make a change. And the use of many approaches across the US will make it difficult to understand GFR change when a patient receives care in different settings or institutions. If you're in Boston and you're at the Beth Israel and you are hospitalized or go to the Brigham three blocks away, your GFR could change, and you could have kidney disease at one institution but not the other. That's a big problem. Some approaches promulgated to remove race, as I showed you, institutionalized discrimination or may be racist. So, the solution should be consistent, durable, evidence-based, and devised with the input of clinicians, system leaders, social scientists, and patients.

Let me leave you with this: what we're trying to achieve is health equity. [Fig. 15] So where should we set our sights? There are huge drivers of disparities. I know that from being involved in this work for nearly 30 years now, and we need to look at all the drivers that are really driving disparities that I showed you and started out with. So, thank you for your attention. I look forward to the discussion.

Moderated Discussion

KIRSTEN BIBBINS-DOMINGO: Thank you very much. I'd like to invite the panelists to join us. Excellent. Thank you, Dr. Grubbs and Dr. Powe, for those outstanding flash talks. I want to invite, first, our additional panelists to each give just one to two minutes reflection on what you've heard. You've each been involved in the debate that both Dr. Grubbs and Dr. Powe laid out so nicely, and I'd love to have you each reflect on it from your perspective. Dr. Adler?

JOSH ADLER: Good morning. Thank you, and I appreciate having the opportunity to participate in this morning and the series. So, as you know, we recently made a change in our eGFR reporting, as Dr. Powe referred to. We discussed many of the elements that Dr. Grubbs and Dr. Powe elucidated thoroughly during the first part of the session. It makes it difficult at the present time for health systems to decide which direction to go, given all of the varying opinions about this issue and the lack, now, of a national standard approach, which really is so important. That said, some of the points were so persuasive that we needed to make a change here at UCSF Health. And so, I very much appreciate the fact that our organization has such expertise and allowed us, unlike many other institutions across the country, to take a step forward, and hopefully a good step forward on this point.

KIRSTEN BIBBINS-DOMINGO: So just to bring everyone up to the point that UCSF Health made, as Dr. Powe alluded to, the decision to take the race factor out of the reporting … and I think Dr. Burchard actually showed your email at the very first session. I know that both Dr. Powe and Dr. Grubbs presented at the committee that made that decision. Dr. Delgado, you are one of the co-chairs of the task force that Dr. Grubbs alluded to that is making a recommendation on this and published your interim report just on Friday. Maybe you can comment on that?

CYNTHIA DELGADO: Sure. I want to say that both talks represent the crux of our debate. And really, salient points made on both sides of the debate are very important and highlight the importance of having this discussion, on having social responsibility with the delivery of health care. And so over the last 10 months, the task force has been really careful to make sure that the decision that's going to be put forth really does have answers to all of those points that were made, whether or not personally for me as a clinician, I truly want to know whether or not there will be consequences before adapting an approach. And so, having that discussion and having that evidence and gathering it really was important for us. One of the discussions said that there were 26 approaches that have been included in our report, and indeed, we do have 26 approaches that we have examined. I think it's important to understand that there are two different things that were that we're thinking about. There's removal of race from the equation and the removal of race from the reporting. Of the 26 approaches, there are 21 approaches that have taken one side or the other. Of those 21 approaches, 10 are creatinine based and 11 are non-creatinine-based approaches. And doing a careful evaluation of which approach would be the best for everyone is important.

KIRSTEN BIBBINS-DOMINGO: Terrific. Dr. Richmond, you've been involved in bringing this to the attention at the forefront of our health systems and certainly involved in this discussion as well. Maybe I can ask you to reflect on the conversation as well.

STEPHEN RICHMOND: Yeah, absolutely. Thank you so much and thank you to our discussants on the matter. I think that, as Dr. Delgado said, it firmly sort of positions us right at the crux of the two sides of where we've been at. I think that there are some grounds that we can stand on that it that is indeed common, which is that we're essentially here for health equity and we're here to achieve what is best for our patients. I do think that there are some significant underpinnings that are complicated and allow for this divide to continue to exist. And in its persistence, a lot of that tension of what has played out for the last 30, 50, 100 years of this country is there and present.

My background is really in critical race theory, I'm not a nephrologist. I'm a family medicine doctor by training. But I often wade into the waters of these discussions on the basis of an understanding of what race is, how race is used, and how it differs from racism especially at the intersection of medicine. I think that I had a lot of thoughts as the two discussants proceeded, one of which is just that if we take a step back and we understand eGFR to be a case study, it is in fact that. It is an individual, not unique, example of what has happened in medicine time and time again and has happened for many years. And so eGFR being a topic that has had the most discussion built up around it, it will serve as a precedent moving forward for how we think about these topics over and over again, whether it be PFTs or ASCVD scores, or feedback calculators. It will be the benchmark in the ways in which we think about this. So again, as Dr. Delgado mentioned, being very careful and thoughtful about the approach is really, really important.

I want to speak to that for a moment, because I feel that we have an opportunity for a turning point here, an opportunity to make a left turn instead of a right turn, instead of repeating past mistakes that have persisted, because of the historical presence of white supremacy in this country. We have an opportunity here to interrupt that process and to do something different, to say that we stood on the right side of history and did so for the right reasons. And so, I think it's challenging when we have this presentation of what feels right because of our training, our education, what feels okay, this is normative, this is the way that we have always followed along in our academic, in our medical, in our clinical practice, to sort of go against that and to stand on something different, to stand on these principles of equity which we often don't do in medicine because they are sort of uninformed by what feels like the right way to evidence. So, I want to make an opportunity in this panel at some point in time to question how our evidence has actually been constructed. We have, for so long, with reckless abandon almost, just given ourselves to evidence – what the evidence shows, what the evidence shows – but not to question how the machine that produces that evidence itself can be biased, itself can improperly route and construct it in the ways in which those results, those interpreters, those clinical practices that result from that contaminated evidence or contaminated process, can produce and reproduce harm over and over and over again. So, I'll leave it at that. I'm sorry to go on, but I do it again appreciate being here and look forward to continuing this conversation with the rest of the discussants.

KIRSTEN BIBBINS-DOMINGO: Great. So, I framed this as a debate and I want to press all of you to try to see the areas that we agree and that this conversation is about what the next step forward is, what we should do tomorrow given the importance of this problem. Or where do we actually have fundamental disagreements? Dr. Grubbs or Dr. Powe?

VANESSA GRUBBS: I'm happy to weigh in on this. I think what is most striking about the two different camps is the camp that wants to maintain or think race is important to keep in our equations all hinges upon there being a biologic difference between the races. And I feel like if we could actually accept that it is not, even though that's what we've been doing since slavery, that we could actually move on to a different way of seeing things. So, to me, there's a lot of conversation about the evidence and who said whatever, but in truth, it's really about a belief system that the different races represent something different biologically. So, to me, that's the only way forward, is for medicine to understand, acknowledge that it really has a problem in upholding white supremacy ideology. And then we can move forward.

KIRSTEN BIBBINS-DOMINGO: Dr. Powe?

NEIL POWE: Yeah, so I would say that we could all agree that, in an ideal world, we wouldn't use this variable called race. But race may be a surrogate for a variety of things, for some social and perhaps even some biological things. But it is a social construct. There is no question about that. But there's something when you look at GFR that race is capturing in terms of the non-GFR determinants of serum creatinine. And so, if that's different and science shows it's different, if we don't use that information to take the best care of our patients, that's not the right thing to do. It's not the use of race. It's the misuse of race. And I think each of these clinical situations – whether it's pulmonary function tests or looking at cognitive function which is very similar to the GFR argument, or GFR, or the indices for cardiac surgery and looking at survival that include race – they're all very, very nuanced and we can't have a blanket approach that says 'just remove it' because you got to have a replacement. And the reason for that replacement is that if you don't look carefully at the evidence, you could do more harm to African Americans than the good that we're all trying to achieve. So, this is very nuanced.

I encourage people to think before they act and to look at all the evidence and particularly, as Dr. Delgado mentioned, the consequences that will happen from different approaches that are taken. I'm in this because I want to do the best for my patients and my minority patients, and I want to use science and evidence to drive that. And I just want to think. I don't want to just have a blanket approach because medicine is more nuanced than that.

KIRSTEN BIBBINS-DOMINGO: Dr. Richmond, you've argued that it's the base of knowledge from which we are deriving these decisions that is in fact problematic, and the way in which we've constructed that base of knowledge. Talk a little bit more about that.

STEPHEN RICHMOND: Yeah, when we think about the misuse, as Dr. Powe had called it, the misuse of race… any sort of assumption or presumption that allows for race to be used or upheld in a way that it's suggested as a sort of biological factor, that there's an underlying biological association, is in fact a misuse. And whether that appears as the sort of current non-Black, or should I say African American or non-African American dichotomy, or a blended equation as Dr. Powe was suggesting, could be served as an appropriate replacement, it still goes back to the same idea of improper categorization of individuals based on a social construct. The idea that an individual could be fully captured – their biology, their exposures, their ancestral history or makeup – could be fully captured in the way that they sort of wake up in the morning and decide to self-identify is, to me, I keep getting this getting back to this … Dr. Powe said you want to think, you want to think, you want to think… and to me, it's the critical thinking that has been obviated from this entire space that has allowed for this exact problem to persist over time.

If you have race, for example, and people identify as Black, white, Hispanic, or other – these are discrete arbitrary categories that essentially started off as socio-political designations, as classifications that were constructed by government as a way of sort of organizing and distributing power, and they continue to be that in this country. And to allow for medicine to be sort of based on that is essentially to further that goal of white supremacy as it is invested and structuralized in this country through racist principles. I'll give you an example. I was reading this article on CNN about politicians in Brazil (this just came out a week ago) and it said that about 43,000 Brazilian politicians changed their racial self-identification from what it was to something different, whether that be white Hispanic, or Black Hispanic or Latino, I should say Latinx, and this has happened over the course of four to five years. Now I want to fully understand – and I'll actually invite Dr. Powe to in respond to this – for those 43,000 politicians that decided overnight, because of political reasons, to change their race, how does medicine see that? How do we hold these individuals in a race conscious way? How do we decide to do something that's accurate and precise for those individuals who have decided, based on their political leanings, to self-identify in a different way now because of the conditions in their sociopolitical environment? What would you do for those individuals?

NEIL POWE: So, if I understand this, you're saying that people may manipulate the reporting of race to their advantage. Did I get that right?

STEPHEN RICHMOND: That's exactly what I'm saying, that people self-identify differently based on environmental factors, based on social factors, based on political factors. That race is something that can change over time whereas biology and ancestry typically is not thought of in that way.

NEIL POWE: Right. So, the way I think of this is that there's a lot of heterogeneity. Race and ethnicity are not the only characteristic that we have. We have geography and ancestry, sex, sexual orientation, sexual identity. I mean, we're a heterogeneous society and even our labels and the way we look at ourselves has changed over time. So, we have to be – and I think you're getting at this – we have to be learning people. And we do have to adapt to the changing definitions. But I think we need to look and say, *is the way that people are applying something the wrong way to apply it or is it a good way?* In fact, people love their identity. I love my identity. I hope this doesn't bother anybody. For the first nine years of my life, I was called a negro and I looked down at myself because I had to fill out that form in school that said negro. Then in 1965, James Brown came out with a record called '*Say it Loud, I'm Black and I'm Proud*' and that was an enormous uplift because it said *my identity can be good, okay? My identity could be good.* And we all have that, no matter what the characteristics we're talking about. And so, the way I look at this is, what are we using any tool of characterizing identity, how are we applying it? And so, we need to do a deep dive and we need to censor the inappropriate application of any identity factor. But we also need to embrace our identity … since I treat… many come to minority physicians and say, "it's great I have a minority physician, so you're going to treat me because of my identity… You know, as a minority physician, what is good for me," and they believe sometimes that different things are better for them or their needs are different.

So, we need to embrace that. We shouldn't just say "oh, we're just going to make this raceless." We need to think, and we need to – if we're engaging patients – we need to ask our patients and share decision-making and education about what we do. And race is not the only the only identity factor here. It's every, all of it, all of it. And that will make us better doctors.

KIRSTEN BIBBINS-DOMINGO: So, let me probe just a little bit. I'd urge you to reflect – and maybe I'm going to ask Dr. Adler and Dr. Delgado to start first – on what we think it means to have a conversation with a patient that sees a different correction or a different number, and the attribution of that different number to their race. What does that mean?

And then, for both of you too, Dr. Delgado and Dr. Adler, you both are representing and acting on behalf of larger organizations. So, what does that mean to make those decisions? We're all individual, as Neil says, and our identities are important. But you're making decisions that affect how we then treat large groups of patients in systematic ways, in different ways. Dr. Adler, would you reflect a little on that?

JOSH ADLER: Sure. So, I think you're actually hitting on why UCSF Health, why would the other organizations that have changed their eGFR reporting, why would they do it in advance of some national new guideline? And I think for us, it was just this point you're making now, which is that although there were many factors considered – many of which were important and relevant to this decision – probably the most important was the degree to which, for our own clinician environment as well as for patients, the continued use of race in the reporting of eGFR clearly contributes to this notion that has been brought up many, many times of race coming from a biological framework rather than a socio-political framework. As an institution, we did not feel that that was right, that that should not be something that we publish, we report on, or we distinguish, let alone the fact that in the age of electronic health records with greater and greater access – in fact most recently, open notes now for all patients across the country – that having a distinction of a test result based on race for our patients with no explanation, but even if there were an explanation, it just is, for the reasons we've just discussed, not the right thing for us all to be doing.

And so even in the absence of a national recommendation, it was that fact that led to the decision to take race out of the reporting at UCSF Health.

KIRSTEN BIBBINS-DOMINGO: Dr. Delgado?

CYNTHIA DELGADO: So, on a national level, both the National Kidney Foundation and the American Society of Nephrology have already come out and said that race is a social not a biological construct and it should be removed from future reporting. On a clinical level, as a nephrologist, you alluded to the question of how does this affect the patient physician relationship and the dialogue you have with your patient. I run the Low Kidney Function Clinic at the San Francisco VA, and I do want to remind everyone that although this topic that we're debating now is really important, when we're talking about kidney function decline and planning for other services that are needed, there's more to the story than just looking at the eGFR report. We look at other parameters related to kidney function decline. It also helps create the dialogue with the patient to decide on what might be the best plan of action, given whatever the patient decides is really important.

Personally, I believe that that's a moment for a dialogue to talk about the accuracy of the equations and whether or not my elderly patient population would have even been included in some of these equation derivations. And at moments when I don't know that the equation is appropriate, I should say that the VA still uses the four variable MDRD and the San Francisco VA does have Cystatin C available. I confirm, but beyond that confirmation, there's also the blood urea nitrogen trend. There's also level of acidosis. There's also how the patient feels. There's been this discussion a little bit alluding on muscle mass. Well, patients who have severe CKD and have kidney function decline have severe muscle atrophy. And at the same time, they have an increase in volume overload. So, using a guide for muscle mass with an estimating equation doesn't seem to gel quite well with the clinical care around patients. So having that dialogue, understanding where the patient wants to be, what's important to them, and then giving them the framework for how you're thinking with the information in front of you is really important. And I really do appreciate this dialogue and the thoughtfulness with which we're all approaching this, because it is important for us to talk about, as Dr. Richmond talked about, the role of race and how this is an inflection point to make a left turn and really lead this country as an organization into dismantling the areas in which race should not be included in clinical decision making.

KIRSTEN BIBBINS-DOMINGO: Thank you. So, one of the most challenging things when we educate new physicians, medical students, any type of clinician, is how we incorporate the fact that we are uncertain about many things into giving them guidance for how to make clinical decisions. And in this case, we have the issues of uncertainty against the larger socio-political backdrop of race and racism in medicine as we've been talking about. So what's your advice to how we should teach about this if you are teaching the medical students? And not the great lectures that you've given, but how would you tell the medical student who's rotating and following you through clinic about whatever version of eGFR is presented in clinic? How would you teach the medical student about how to approach this particular topic in the clinical decisions as they're learning to take care of a patient?

VANESSA GRUBBS: I'd like to weigh in on this because this is something that I have been doing during my 10 years of being on faculty at San Francisco General and running our version of the clinic that Dr. Delgado is speaking of for patients with advanced chronic kidney disease. What I would tell them is, I would explain to them where this whole 'if African-American' thing came from and explain to them that supposedly it was a proxy for muscle mass. It wasn't really backed up by much, so we need to be much more thoughtful about it. It's not just about the race of the person, because clearly what we can see for patients who are approaching end-stage kidney disease – they are losing muscle mass. And as I presented, I think the problem with only suggesting that race is the deciding factor is really problematic and inaccurate for all the patients, not just the Black patients.

And I have never encountered a student – or a resident for that matter, and not even some of the neurology fellows –aware of this background. So, I think this really just shows us how entrenched our beliefs about race can be, that nobody bothers to question it because this is the way it is, this is the way it's always been, and everybody's doing it this way without really being thoughtful about it. And when the conversation talks about 'this is a very nuanced thing', I question who is it nuanced for? Because it's lumping all Black people together and suggesting that all Black people are fundamentally different than everybody else on the planet without any real explanation. I mean, as I've written and spoken about before, nephrology is supposed to be this field of real precision. And yet, when it comes to kidney function, 'if you think you're Black', that's the only decision point rather than thinking about whether or not people are vegan, whether or not people are bodybuilders, what particular medications they're taking… And these are all the things that really affect when we're talking about creatinine, the production of creatinine, and how the kidneys clear it.

KIRSTEN BIBBINS-DOMINGO: Thank you. Anyone else want to weigh in on how you would explain this to the medical students who are trying to make the decision for how to approach this for a patient?

CYNTHIA DELGADO: Well, I'd like to weigh in with Dr. Grubbs. I generally agree with the same approach, and I generally use the same exact approach with talking about kidney function. But I also make sure that the trainees are aware that the estimating equation is based on measured GFR and the measured GFR is done by iothalamate or iohexol. It's not a perfect science. It's not an inulin clearance. We don't exactly have a gold standard that is exactly perfect to estimate the exact, to know what the exact kidney function is for any one individual. So, for me, the estimating estimated GFR is based on a measured GFR that's also estimated. So, it's an estimate of an estimate.

And so definitely the dialogue about the inclusion of all the coefficients and the issues and the flaws with the equations themselves, including the use of race, are important and should be brought up as quickly as we can with our trainees to talk about and have this dialogue about how to quickly, critically examine this and put this in perspective. I do think that there's more to having a dialogue about kidney function estimation and kidney function decline then looking at an eGFR and saying, 'oh this person's eGFR is 20, you got to start dialysis.' You have someone in front of you who may be feeling fine and may not necessarily fit that box that you're thinking about and it's really critically important for us to use medicine as a guide rather than an absolute.

VANESSA GRUBBS: If I could just add that I think the underlying point here is that race, the inclusion of race, gives us this perception that we're somehow getting more precise and more helpful for this group of people when it really isn't doing that at all. And the measured GFR might be somewhere 30% higher and 30% percent lower than the estimated GFR. I think we're really doing a disservice to our trainees by teaching them that you're losing something, that you're doing something wrong, if you don't consider the race of the person. I'll leave it there.

KIRSTEN BIBBINS-DOMINGO: Thank you. Dr. Adler?

JOSH ADLER: Yeah, I just wanted to pick up a little bit on this point about precision. Drs. Grubbs and Delgado are speaking in many ways as experts in kidney disease, but most of the creatinines and eGFR's are interpreted by non-experts in kidney disease. And so, one of the goals of the change at UCSF Health was to increase the feelings of uncertainty about this test a little bit, to engender more discussion, whether it's with patients or with trainees about what the 'e' in eGFR even means. It means estimate. And so we need to be more serious about the fact that this is only an estimate so that other factors that have been described many times can be considered, including by the way, the use of Cystatin C. So just wanted to mention that that was one of the goals we were trying to achieve was to increase at least consideration for the use of Cystatin C. And we've seen about a threefold increase in the use of Cystatin C since making the change here. Now whether the clinical decisions are correct based on those uses, we don't know yet. But certainly, there's more there's more seeking for clarity, I think, as a result of this.

KIRSTEN BIBBINS-DOMINGO: Great. Dr. Richmond, did you have something else?

STEPHEN RICHMOND: Yeah, I did. Thank you. So, I just wanted to speak to your question more specifically, Dr. Domingo, around education. I just wanted to give a huge shout out to students and trainees who have been on the front lines of this issue. I want to be careful to understand that one of the reasons why we are having this discussion, this series, and one of the reasons why this movement has taken national visibility is because medical students and trainees who are the ones that are supposed to be being educated are the ones who have called this into question to begin with. They are the ones who are oftentimes having to figure out how to strategically teach up and ask these critical questions that have historically locked us into the space of structuralized racism in medicine. They're the ones that are trying to figure out 'okay how do I exist in this space exhausted every day with this confronted with this onslaught of microaggressions every single day', which GFR may in fact be one of them, and say, 'okay I want to bring this up to my attending. I want to question this' and then they get essentially smacked down. And that's just the way it is.

This is what the evidence shows. So, I just want to be careful to remember that part of our change and evolution on this is realizing that teaching comes from all directions. And so the question could equally be asked: What are the ways in which medical students can be invited to teach up to their attendings? What are the ways in which they can be heard? What are the ways in which this can be more well received in these discussions, which complicate and interrupt white supremacy as usual, can be welcomed into the academic space? I don't know where we would be in this space without, for example, students at the Institute of Healing & Justice in Medicine, who have led this discussion nationally, who have essentially taught and done so much in instruction and invitation on organizing and helped lead the way for folks at University of Washington or Vanderbilt or NGH. But there's just been so much work that has been done in the ground level that has been essentially unheard, quieted, unspoken while administrators and institutions have looked as the vanguards in this space around leading change. So, I just wanted to give a big shout out to the medical students and trainees who are really doing the work on the ground.

KIRSTEN BIBBINS-DOMINGO: Thank you, Dr. Richmond. Dr. Powe, would you come up, too, on teaching the medical student who's shadowing you on clinic or on the wards?

NEIL POWE: Sure, and I would do this for anything. I would say, what clinical decision are you trying to solve? And once we honed in on that, then we should use the evidence to help guide us. Let me give an example. So, in this case, I'm trying to think about how to dose a drug – let's say chemotherapy for a Black woman with ovarian cancer. I picked that because it's been shown that Black women are less likely to receive adequate doses of carboplatin therapy. That's been very demonstrated. So, if I give them the non-Black eGFR, then that will just exacerbate that. And already, it's exacerbated because we use non-indexed GFR, often, to dose drugs when we should be… well, we use indexed GFR rather than non-indexed GFR. We know that many African American women are overweight or obese, which adds to the problem of inadequate dosing. So, this just exacerbates the under treatment.

And then if you go to transplant waitlisting, one of the fallacies is the problem is we make use of these thresholds – eGFR less than 20, that's the trigger for a referral. That's what I call equality. What if we turn this around and said equity? Then you would say, because African Americans progress faster, they have a greater need and it's need that we want to get at. Then you would get rid of that equality threshold, and you would give African Americans, and I have to say other racial minorities, what they need. So, we are fixated on these numbers and these algorithms that we need to think and restructure even the way that we allocate resources and how we do that.

When it comes to giving someone a drug, I want to be as careful as I can because that could a life or a death decision. So could getting a transplant. But I have a little bit more time to think about that. And what's great at UCSF Health is that you get two values, you can use either of those values to put people over that threshold if they're borderline on the threshold. And I think that's what people are speaking to about the uncertainty and then how we use the data. So that's what I would do. I would teach the medical student to be the advocate for their patient, both on the access side but also on the biology side and the medical side about how to best treat the patient. That's what it's all about and it's not just a trigger. It's thinking about it, thinking about the patient, as Dr. Delgado said, all the issues that you think about in making a specific clinical decision.

KIRSTEN BIBBINS-DOMINGO: Thank you. Thank you very much. This has been a really terrific panel. I really appreciate Dr. Powe and Dr. Grubbs laying out the important issues here as well as the discussion of what this means for how we take care of patients, how in our systems we make decisions for how we do the best for all of our patients.

Case Study 3: Race, Genetic Ancestry, and Disease Risk Flash Talks

KIRSTEN BIBBINS-DOMINGO: We're now going to turn to our last case study, and this is going to begin with a video followed by two flash talks given by Professor Ryan Hernandez, who is an Associate Professor of Bioengineering in the UCSF School of Medicine and School of Pharmacy. He's a population geneticist that will be followed by a Dr. Elad Ziv, who is a Professor of Medicine, a general internist, and a physician scientist studying cancer genetics.

This will be followed by a panel of discussion, one our two flash talk speakers will join, a panel moderated by a Professor Aimee Medeiros, who is Associate Professor of History of Health Sciences in the UCSF School of Medicine and a member of our steering committee for this session. She'll be joined by Dr. Denise Connor, who is a physician and educator at UCSF and leads our anti-oppression curriculum, Dr. Shoumita Dasgupta, who is a Professor and Assistant Dean at Boston University, geneticist, and educator, and Dr. Aleksander Rajkovic, who is the Chief Genomics Officer at UCSF. So, we'll begin with the video.

NARRATOR: Polygenic risk scores are numbers used to estimate the effect of many genetic variants on an individual's risk for disease. They are used to predict the risk of complex diseases, such as breast cancer, prostate cancer, and diabetes, which are caused by an interplay of environmental and behavioral factors with the particular genetic variants that a person inherited. Polygenic risk scores have been shown to predict the risk of some chronic diseases more accurately than current clinical models. However, polygenic risk scores currently have far greater predictive value in individuals of European descent than groups with other ancestries, which presents a major challenge to equitable implementation of precision medicine. Here, we show an example from breast cancer.

Thousands of individuals' genomes were analyzed for genetic variants associated with breast cancer. They were then stratified into percentiles based on the number of risk variants they had. From this data, we could estimate the lifetime risk of developing breast cancer tailored to an individual's particular genetic makeup. So, how do polygenic risk scores work? Each of us has a genome composed of approximately 3 billion nucleotide base pairs, or the letters of DNA, that spell out about 20,000 genes and shape who we are. But the vast majority of our genomes are identical. Only about 0.1 percent of the base pairs in our genomes differ among individuals, and these variants are referred to as single nucleotide polymorphisms, or SNPs. These SNPs account for the genetic differences among us, such as eye color, height, and even our risk for certain diseases. Most of the SNPs in an individual's genome are shared across all human populations, but due to our unique patterns of human migration and ancestry, some of them are found more commonly in one population while others are rare and only ever found in a particular population.

SNPs that are close together on a chromosome are often inherited together in a block, so even though the SNP we actually detect might not be causing the variation we see, we can predict it will be inherited along with the causal SNP. SNPs can be easily detected at a very low cost by a process called genotyping. This has allowed us to analyze SNPs from millions of people to look for associations between these SNPs and whether or not people have certain diseases such as breast cancer, prostate cancer, diabetes, and hypertension. This type of study is called a genome-wide association study. For complex diseases, individual SNPs often contribute only a tiny increased risk of disease. However, some people carry many disease-associated SNPs and may have elevated genetic risk for that disease. This is the idea behind polygenic risk scores.

We can estimate a person's risk of disease by summing up all the genetic risk factors they carry in their genome. So, how well do polygenic risk scores work across different populations? Well, polygenic risk scores derived from one global population typically perform much worse in other populations. For example, one study found that polygenic risk scores based on study participants from Japan were less accurate when applied to British people of European or African ancestry and vice versa. There are many possible reasons for this.

First, SNPs and inheritance blocks can differ significantly between populations based on their genetic history. So, if we want to estimate genetic risk for a disease in a different population, we need to study that population directly. Second, differences in behavior and the environment across populations can affect how predictive genetic variants are in determining disease risk. What is a population? Globally, humans form a continuum of genetic ancestry connecting all of us from our evolutionary origins in Africa through waves of migration spreading across the world. Race and ethnicity are social constructs that seek to simplify the complex relationships among all humans on the basis of physical characteristics and cultural heritage, respectively.

In contrast, genetic ancestry is a measure of similarity among individuals based on their genetic variants and is most closely related to the geographic origins of the individual's ancestors. Race and ethnicity can be correlated to genetic ancestry, but they are not the same. Therefore, race and ethnicity are better predictors of social determinants of health, such as exposure to racism, while ancestry is a better predictor of genotype. Unfortunately, the human genetics community has not done a great job of studying the continuum of human populations. Approximately 80 percent of all genome-wide association study participants are of European descent, despite making up only 16 percent of the global population. From a genetic perspective that means we're missing a lot of the global genetic variation.

And from a healthcare perspective, we run the risk of exacerbating health disparities. This is because the polygenic risk scores we derive are less accurate in underrepresented populations and thus the benefits are not evenly distributed. To fix this, we need to include populations of diverse ancestries. However, because genetic ancestry is determined by genotyping, we first need to recruit people based on self-defined social constructs of race and ethnicity as proxies for underlying genetic variation. Thus, to improve diversity in genetic ancestry, studies need to improve racial and ethnic diversity. When we do so, we can improve polygenic risk scores for everyone.

For example, the inclusion of a large number of men of African ancestry in a recent study improved the precision of polygenic risk scores for predicting prostate cancer risk in both European and African populations. Moving forward, we need to prioritize the inclusion of diverse populations in genomic research and to better understand the impact of environmental factors.

These steps will improve the value of polygenic risk scores for non-European populations and advance equity and genomic health for all.

KIRSTEN BIBBINS-DOMINGO: Excellent. Dr. Hernandez?

A Population Genetics View on Race and Ancestry

Ryan Hernandez, PhD

RYAN HERNANDEZ: Wonderful. Thank you so much for the opportunity. I wanted to talk today about the basic science of thinking about race, ethnicity and ancestry coming at this from a population genetics perspective. My real interest is in understanding the phenotypic variation that we see across the world. There is a tremendous amount of phenotypic variation within the global human population, and it's largely thought that much of this phenotypic variation has to do with our evolutionary history. As a species, we evolved within Africa some 200,000 years ago and, over the last several thousand years, have finally colonized the entire world. And what's amazing about this is that it's only within the last 10- to 15- thousand years is that humans have been the only homo species on earth. Throughout our evolutionary history, there have been many homo species that have coexisted, but only within the last 10- to 15- thousand years have we become the only homo species. And that's remarkable, and it owes to thinking about how we consider humans as a species and as a population. But as humans have migrated across the population, not necessarily everybody has moved from one location to another. Obviously, many people stay behind.

We can think about how those migrations and movements across the world affect human populations and the genetic patterns we see in different human populations. I like to think about human genetics as an urn full of a bunch of different genetic variants. [Fig. 1] You can imagine this is a population of genomes and each of these different colored balls represent different patterns of genetic variation. If only a small number of people move from one location in the world to another, it's like taking a small sample of the genetic variation that exists in that prior population. And so, we end up with a small number of individuals representing just a small fraction of the genetic variation that existed in the previous population. But, of course, that population typically grows – they find a new niche, they find a new environment that they can thrive in, new resources that they can access, and that population grows. But

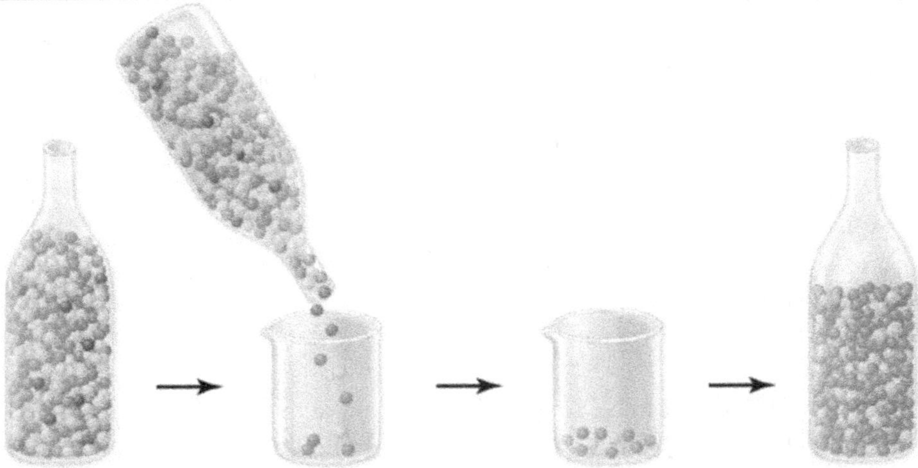

Fig. 1

when that population grows, the genetic diversity within that population grows slowly. All mutations that enter enter in as very rare variants within a population. It takes a long time for those mutations to increase in frequency. So, what we see is that, in a new population, the genetic variation is a subset of the genetic variation that existed in the previous population. And you can imagine, as humans evolved within Africa and slowly spread and radiated across the world, this resulted in a series of these processes occurring. These processes are called bottlenecks – population bottlenecks – where populations go through sort of a reduction in population size but then expand again to a much larger population size later. And this process has resulted in patterns of genetic variation that are quite different in different regions of the world. [Fig. 2]

This is a plot looking at 2,500 individuals from the 1000 Genomes Project that was published a number of years ago where we're looking at the number of variant sites per genome, and each one of these little points is an individual from a different population, from a different country or a different sampling location. And what we see is that in Africa and many different individuals from different populations in Africa, there tends to be 4.6 to about 5 million variants per individual genome. But if we look at non-African populations, it tends to be much lower – between 4 and 4.2 million variants per individual. And so, given all of this data, given these millions of variants and the different patterns that we see across different number of areas, that we see across different populations, and different combinations that we see across

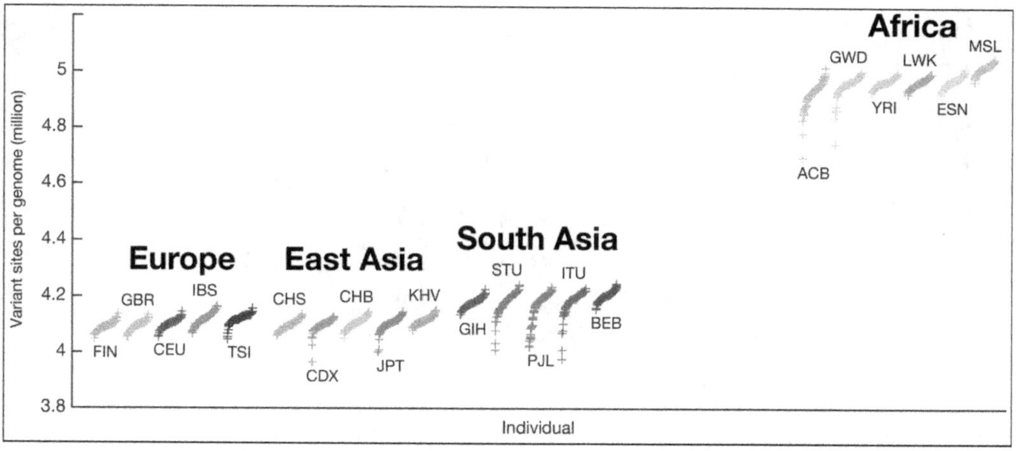

Fig. 2

different populations, it turns out that we can use this information across the genome to stratify different population groups. [Fig. 3] So, if we take a sample of individuals from a European population (this is a group of European ancestry individuals from Utah), if we take a group of individuals sampled from Nigeria, if we take a group of individuals that are identified as Native American, and we look across the genomes, we can use modern tools such as principal component analysis (which is what this represents) to identify different clusters of human populations.

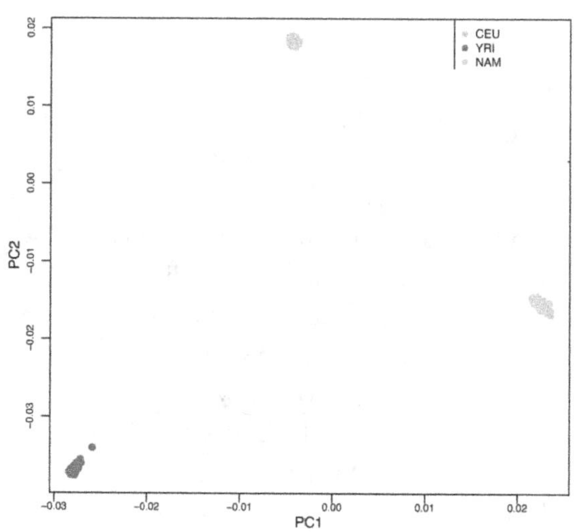

Fig. 3

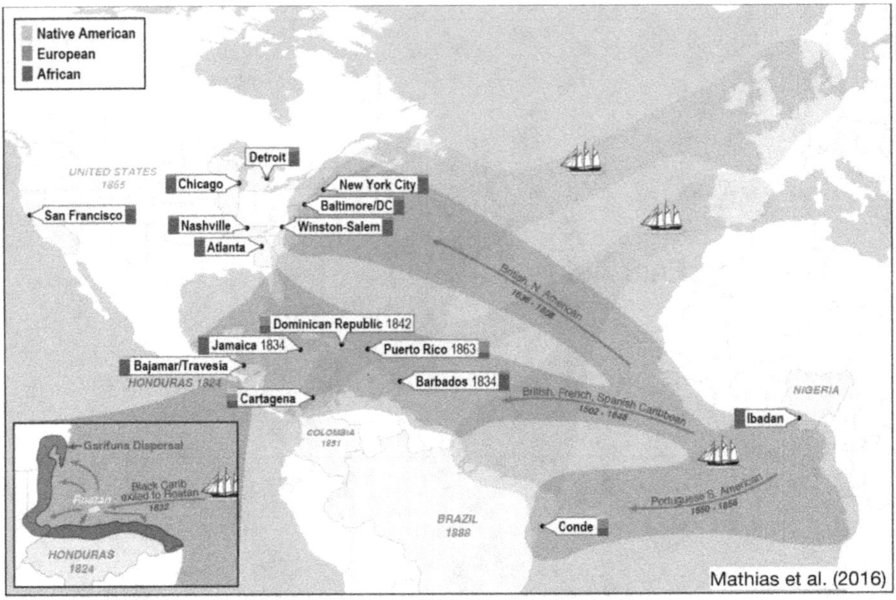

Fig. 4

But, of course, this is a simplistic view of what populations look like in the United States. [Fig. 4] In the United States, we have populations that are characterized by the forced migration of individuals from Africa and the colonization of the United States and the Americas by individuals from Europe, which has resulted in extensive amount of admixture amongst many different populations. And when we look at populations that are sampled within the United States or within the Americas, what we see is that the number of genetic variants in these populations from Peru, Colombia, from Puerto Rico, from African Americans from the southwest, we see a very wide range in the number of genetic variants per genome. And this largely reflects the different ancestries that these individuals have within their genomes.

And so, the way that this works is you can imagine that there's two individuals – an individual from one population from one region of the world and another individual from a different population from a different region of the world. And if they mate and have an offspring, individual from population one will provide a red chromosome to their offspring, and individual from population two will provide a blue chromosome. But, if we have mating within individuals that are that are admixed, then they don't pass on an entire red or blue chromosome anymore. They practice on a recombinant chromosome, which will be partially red and partially blue. And as this process continues over

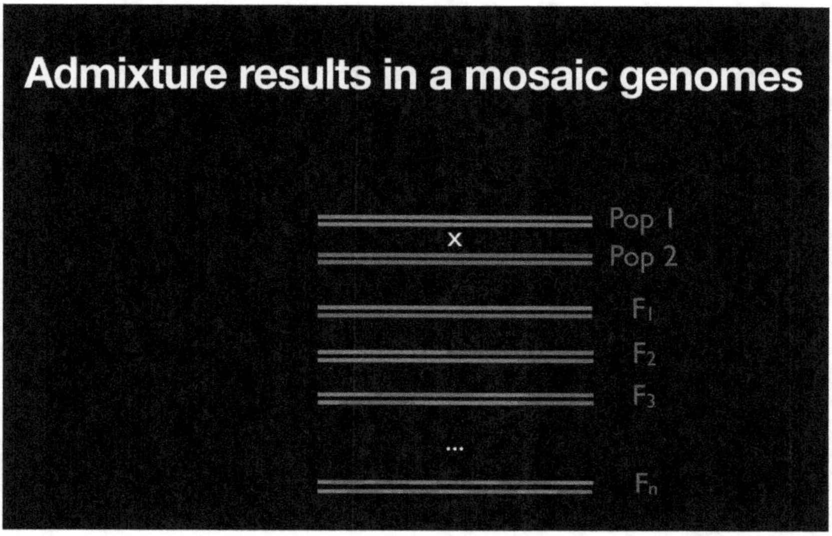

Fig. 5

time, what we end up with is a mosaic of genomes. [Fig. 5] Just an example, I'll show you one. This is me. [Fig. 6] This is my genome from 23andMe, and what you can see is that my ancestry is roughly 70%-71% European, about 20.5% Native American or Amerindigenous, as I like to as I prefer to refer to it, and about 3.6% Sub-Saharan African. And these are distributed across my entire genome.

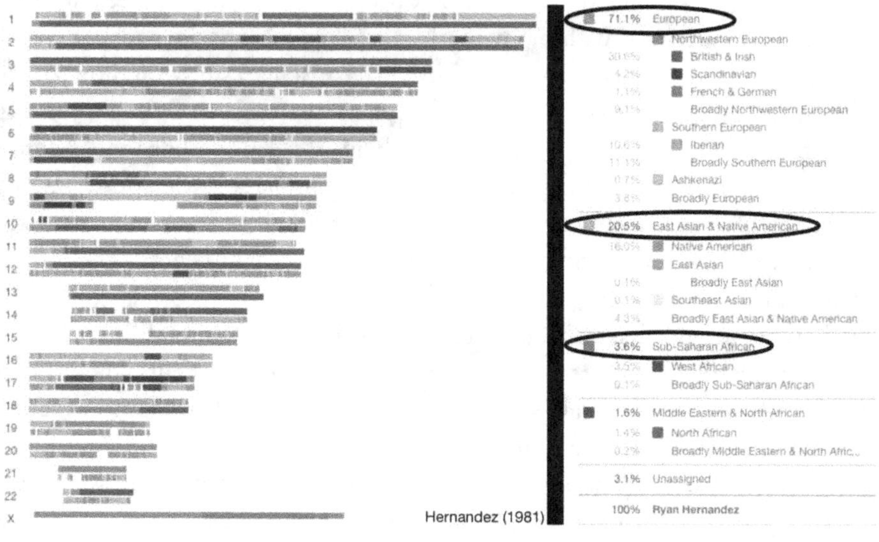

Fig. 6

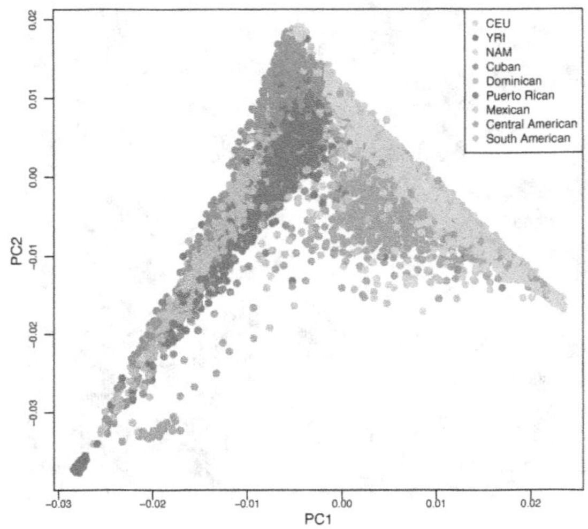

Spear et al (2020)

Fig. 7

And when we look across populations of the US, this admixture process has actually resulted in a continuum of populations. [Fig. 7] We don't have discrete groups that that represent just one population. All of our different population groups are connected through individuals that have varying degrees of ancestry from European, African, and Amerindigenous sources as well as other Asian sources. And it turns out that a lot of these ancestry patterns are correlated with biomedical traits. [Fig. 8, opposite page] So, we've looked within Mexican Americans, in this particular study, at how much the biomedical trait is correlated with ancestry patterns, in this case looking specifically at the degree to which an individual's Amerindigenous ancestry varies. And what we find is that there are some dramatic correlations ranging from height, which is very negatively correlated with Amerindigenous ancestry – the more Amerindigenous ancestry you contain in your genome the shorter you tend to be on average – all the way up to positively correlated factors, such as our friend that we've been discussing this morning, eGFR. And what we notice is that if ancestry is correlated with biomedical traits, then this is potentially something that we really need to access if we're going to think about the care of individuals in our society.

And just to think about the consequences of this idea where we have a human genetics and clinical operation that has been largely biased towards sampling individuals of European ancestry, I want to look specifically at the

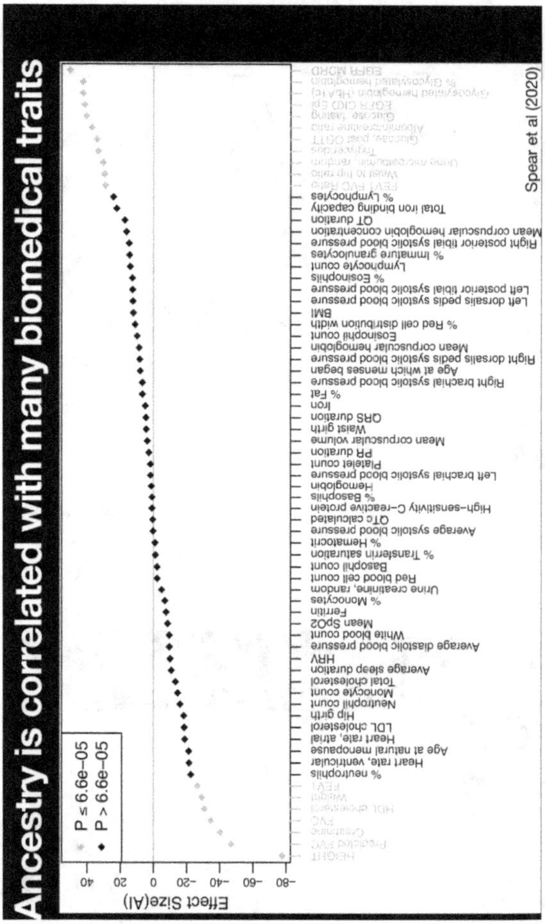

case of height. [Fig. 9] Height is one of the simplest phenotypes to collect. Everybody has one and it's very easy to access, and there are very large samples that have been studied – 300,000 plus individuals from the U.K. Biobank, for example, in with individuals of European ancestry. And we've developed polygenic risk scores or polygenic height scores that that we can use based on these European individuals and ask how well they apply in other populations. We applied it to Mexican Americans in particular, and we asked how well does this polygenic height score work?

Well, it turns out for individuals that are Mexican Americans that have very high levels of European ancestry and very low levels of Amerindigenous ancestry, it actually works quite well. The correlation between their predicted height score and their actual height is highly correlated, p-value of 10^{-5}. However, if you take individuals in the upper quartile for Amerindigenous ancestry or lower quartile for European ancestry, it doesn't work well at all. We have p-values that are greater than 0.08, and in fact, for this other quartile, it's a p-value of 0.6. The predicted height does not correlate with observed height at all. [Fig. 10]

And so, what we have in the United States is that admixtures produced a continuum of populations, and race and ethnicity are really imperfect partitions of this continuum. It's important to point out that more information is actually needed on family history to overcome the systemic underrepresentation of historically excluded groups. And it's important to note that this idea of identifying individuals as white or Black or African American

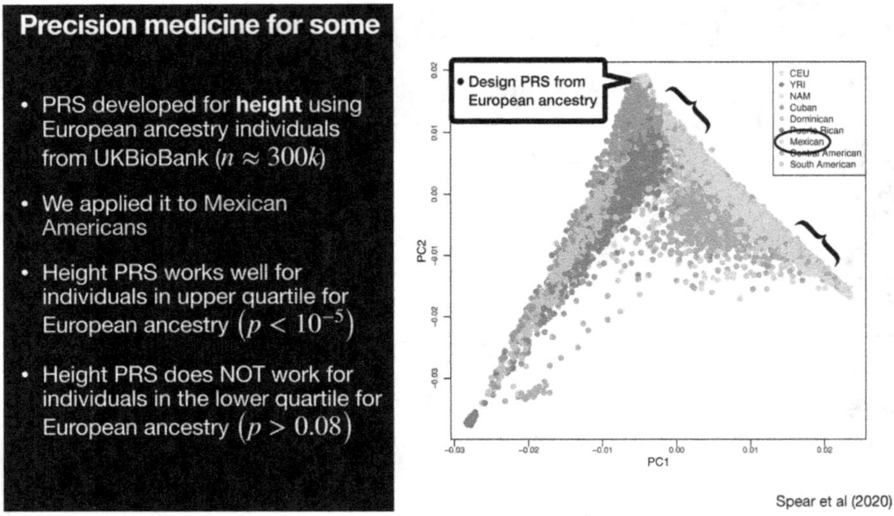

Fig. 9

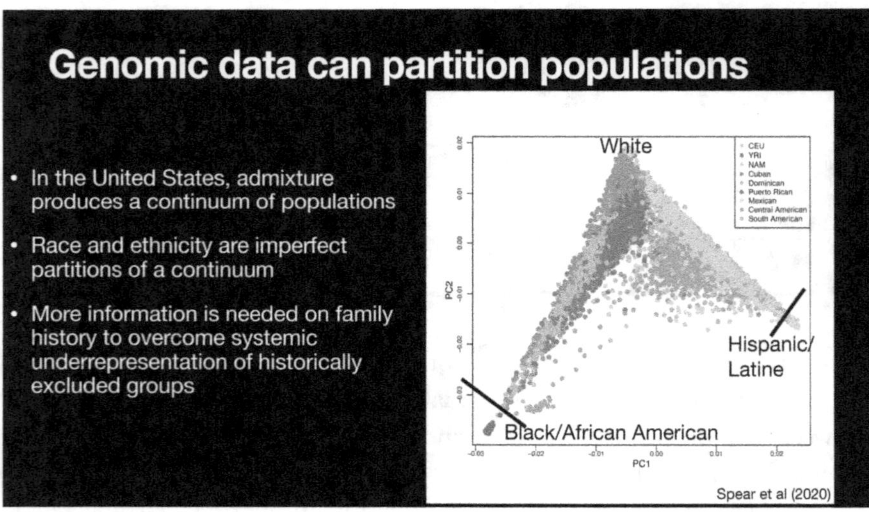

Fig. 10

or Hispanic/Latine is somewhat challenging because all of the individuals that were included in the study are from Hispanic health studies and all of these individuals have self-identified as Hispanic/Latino, some of whom have very high African ancestry, some of whom have very high Amerindigenous ancestry, some of whom have very high European ancestry. But all of these individuals self-identify as Hispanic/Latino. Thank you.

How to Avoid Structural Racism in Precision Medicine: The Case of Polygenic Risk for Breast Cancer

Elad Ziv, MD

ELAD ZIV: Great, thank you for inviting me. I'm going to try and frame this a little bit more in a clinical domain and ask the question of how we use polygenic risk scores and how does that intersect with race and with ancestry, and I'm going to be particularly focusing on the example of polygenic risk or for breast cancer. So, it was already introduced in the introductory video that polygenic risk for breast cancer has been developed, and in fact this slide demonstrates the estimated lifetime risk for women with different polygenic risk score where the top line the orange line represents the top 1 percentile of polygenic risk. [Fig. 1, top] This was a paper published by the Breast Cancer Association Consortium. Unfortunately, what we didn't say is that this is a paper done by European consortium and all of the samples included here are European ancestry. So, the question then is how do we use this in clinical practice?

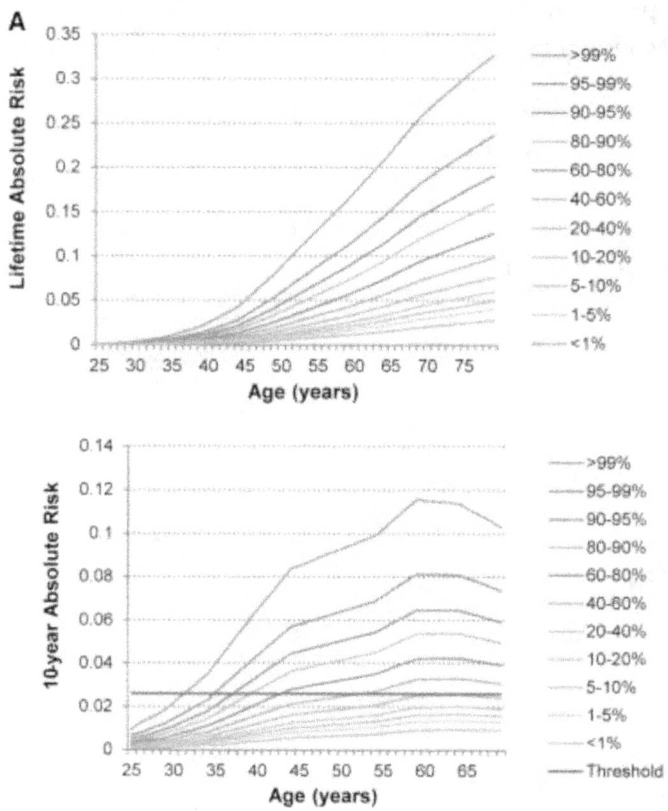

Fig. 1

So, one of the ways we could potentially use in clinical practice is sort of thinking about the onset of screening. So, for example, this is a study done by the U.K. group. [see Fig. 1, bottom] In the U.K., screening starts at age 50 and the average 10-year risk – so this slide demonstrates a 10-year risk by the percentile of polygenic risk scores – the average 10-year risk for a 50-year-old woman is about 2.5%. You can see that the middle line – the blue line there – crosses the threshold at 2.5%. But what you can also see is that there are lots of women, based on their polygenic risk score, who cross that line much earlier. For example, in the 60th to 80th percentile, there are women crossing that threshold on average at age 43, and the top 1 percentile crosses by the time they're actually age 40, which is when we begin to think about screening in the United States. Those women are actually up at about 6% risk. So, you can think that this potentially makes sense to at least consider in the context of screening. This has generated a lot of enthusiasm from some geneticists and possibly some clinicians. I do want to caution that this is sort of all an idea. We haven't really used this. We haven't really shown that it's effective.

So, I'm going to tell you a little bit about the WISDOM trial, which is a one example of how polygenic risk score is being used. [Fig. 2] The WISDOM trial is a trial of breast cancer screening and it's really a comparison of standard screening, which the trial defines as annual mammography starting at age 40.

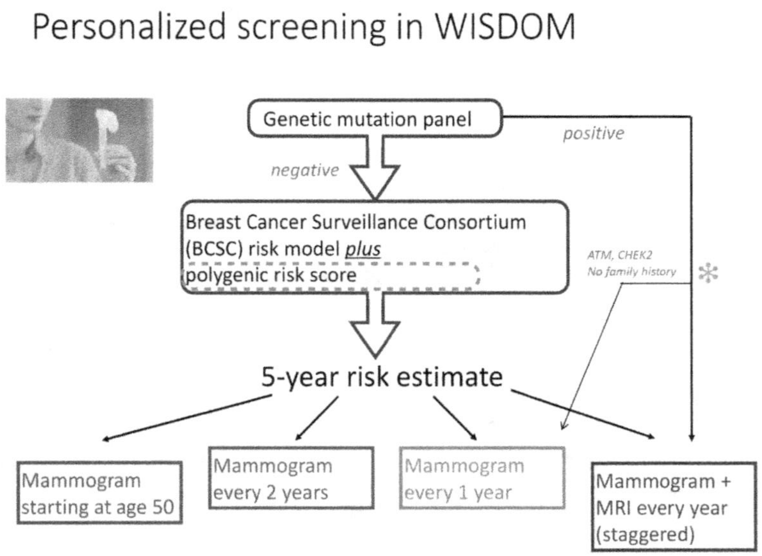

Fig. 2

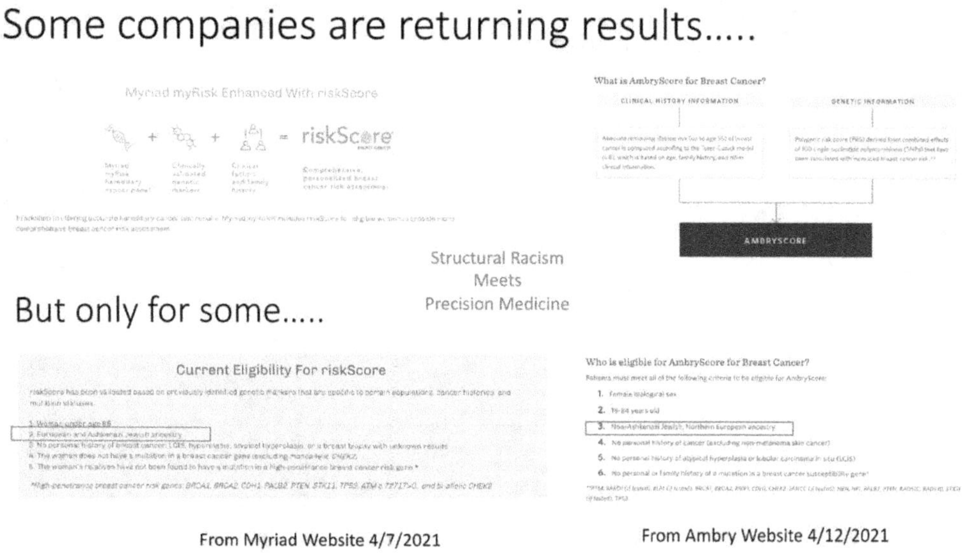

Fig. 3

That is the guideline recommendations by the American College of Radiology and some other institutions. And the comparison group is what is being called the precision or personalized screening arm in the WISDOM trial. And that arm includes a genetic mutation panel testing, so they test for nine breast cancer susceptibility genes. And then women who are positive then get shuffled over to a high-risk screening regimen that includes mammography and MRI every year. And women who either have intermediate penetrance genes (ATM and CHEK2) or women who don't who test negative go into a larger group and are risk stratified, get a polygenic risk model as well as a risk model calculated by the breast cancer surveillance consortium model and get put into bins with the lowest risk women starting mammography at age 50, and then intermediate risk women starting at age in their 40s and getting mammography every year, higher risk women getting mammography every year, and in the highest risk women getting mammogram and MRI every year. So, that's the idea. And as you can see, polygenic risk is part of that. And so, this is an example I think, where we're using this today in a clinical trial setting. We don't know the answer yet, but should this work, then what we would like to do is take this polygenic risk and apply it in the clinic. And the question is, can we? And as I think some of the other speakers have already hinted, it's not going to be

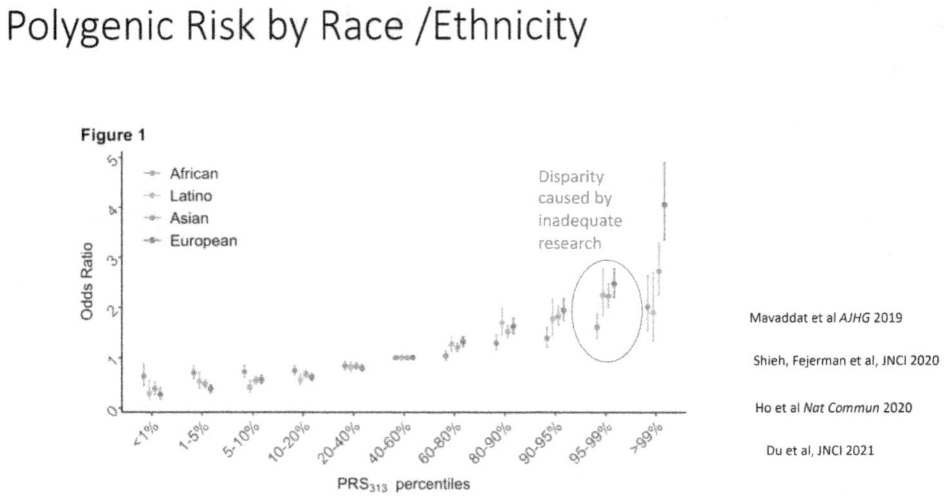

Fig. 4

straightforward based on ancestry.

I just want to say one other thing that, in the clinical domain, some companies are now returning polygenic risk scores. [Fig. 3] So, these are two companies – two of the larger genetic testing companies – and they test for BRCA1, BRCA2, ATM, and CHK2, two other susceptibility genes. If you come back negative, they offer these breast cancer polygenic risk scores. They are returned, but there's a catch. The catch is you have to be a certain age, they're returned only to women, and they say explicitly on their websites that they only return the results if you are a certain ancestry. They particularly say European ancestry. One of them says Ashkenazi Jewish. One of them says non-Ashkenazi Jewish. But the bottom line here is that a large fraction of the US population is not getting the results back, and the question here is what's happening? And I think the one thing I want to say is, we've talked a lot about disparities and the goal of making medicine more equitable. Well, here is an example of where we've actually introduced a disparity. And let me sort of take you through a little bit more of the evidence. I think in some ways, they've been overly restrictive, but the data have probably lagged and they're just coming in now.

So, this is these are some of the data. [Fig. 4] This is actually compiled, as you can see, from four different papers. The 2019 paper by Mavaddat was the polygenic risk score in the European ancestry populations, and then our

Confluence

Table 2: Race/ancestry distribution of non-carrier female breast cancer cases

Race/Ancestry Group	New Genotyping	%	Existing GWAS	%	Total	%
White	91,834	73.3%	144,195	79.1%	236,029	76.7%
Asian	9,803	7.8%	14,068	7.7%	23,871	7.8%
Black or African American	6,670	5.3%	16,508	9.1%	23,178	7.5%
Hispanic or Latina	11,781	9.4%	7,488	4.1%	19,269	6.3%
Unknown	4,324	3.4%			4,324	1.4%
Other	813	0.6%			813	0.3%
American Indian or Alaska Native	109	0.1%			109	<0.1%
Native Hawaiian/Pacific Islander	18	<0.1%			18	<0.1%
TOTAL	125,352		182,259		307,611	

From NCI website

Fig. 5

own paper led by Yiwey Shieh and Laura Fejerman on polygenic risk score in Latinas, a polygenic risk score in Asians by Ho et al., and a polygenic risk score in African Americans and other African ancestry populations was just published by Du et al. And this is sort of compiling all of the results, and you can see on the *x*-axis are the percentile of a polygenic risk score. On the *y*-axis are the odds ratios. And so, what you want to see is sort of a spread. You want to see that the highest risk women are at the highest risk and the lowest risk women are at the lowest risk. And what you're seeing is that it does work, but it works differentially. And in particular, what we're seeing is that if we just take this top – the 95 to 99 percentile group – the polygenic score in the European ancestry women, is about two-and-a-half-fold higher risk compared to the median. In Asian populations, it's 2.2. In Latinas, it's about 2.2. And in the African ancestry population, it's about 1.6. So, half of the predictive power has been lost, and this may be sort of what's been driving this differential reporting on the part of the companies.

The next question is how did we get here. So, this is the largest genome-wide association studies. [Fig. 5] This is actually taken from the NCI website. They're actually running a new genomic association study and you can see the existing genomic association data in the middle panel here. And what you can see is that we've basically been systematically underrepresenting the Black or African American women, also the Asian and Latina women compared to the

Race Conscious Genetics Research

- We need to be aware of the difference between ancestry and race when we analyze studies (and in the clinical domain)
- But we also need to use race to recruit participants BECAUSE we need diverse ancestry in genetic studies
- Otherwise we will get genetic results that will not work well across ancestry groups
- Which will predominantly affect minority populations
- Leading to structural racism in how precision medicine is applied

Fig. 6

European ancestry population. So, 144,000 cases have been GWASed whereas in the Asian, it's 14,000, African American it's been about 16,000. I should say these are data that are existing. They haven't quite been published, so things will get better probably in the near future in the African American population. And even lower sample size in Latinas. And I should add that there are other populations that have really been dramatically underrepresented here. And so, the assumption perhaps was that it'll just work regardless of your ancestry and the result is clearly that it's not. It's working a little bit – better than not at all. But we're losing a lot of information, and this could have implications for the way precision medicine is ultimately applied in different populations.

So, I think the take-home messages I want to impress on you is that we need to be aware of the differences between ancestry and race when we analyze studies. [Fig. 6] And certainly, in the clinical domain, we really need to think about that. But we also need to use race to recruit participants because we need diverse ancestry and genetic studies. If we don't do that, we run the race that the genetic results that we get will not work well across ancestry groups, which will predominantly affect minority populations. And in my view, that leads to a form of structural racism that the precision medicine tools that we're developing that are being paid for by public funds for the most part, by taxpayers, are not going to work well across populations. And I'll stop there.

KIRSTEN BIBBINS-DOMINGO: Great. Thank you very much. And I now want to invite our panelists to come. And just to make a comment that we've chosen both of these case studies today because they represent tools that – eGFR and polygenic risk scores – diagnostic tools that we are either actively using and have used for many years or are on the brink of potentially being used clinically. And both raise issues related to how we should think about race/racism in medicine and the application or the knowledge base that underlies them in the application of clinical practice. So, looking forward to the discussion and I want to turn it over to Dr. Medeiros.

Moderated Discussion

AIMEE MEDEIROS: Thank you so much. Before I turn it to the panelists to give some of their initial feedback, I'd like to provide a little historical context as a historian of medicine. Yesterday, I was reminded by Dr. Denise Davis that history is present. Not only am I compelled to thank Dr. Davis for this reminder, but I would also like to use it as a possible framework for our discussion today about the use of genetic ancestry in medical research and healthcare. In doing so, I'd like to refer back to Dr. Grubbs' comments about the history and legacy of eugenics and medicine.

Eugenics is the practice of, or advocacy for, selective breeding to advance society by championing the reproduction of the fit and eliminating the unfit. The fit category was often seen along racial lines. Elite whites were deemed desirable, and poor whites, the disabled, and people of color were not. In the US, one of the most influential eugenicists was Charles Davenport, a prominent early 20th century biologist. In the 1900s, he became the Director of the Biological Laboratory at Cold Spring Harbor, where he oversaw the collection of data and "inheritable traits" by field workers. While there are fundamental differences between the collection and processing of data by eugenicists then and geneticists and medical researchers now, this history is present with us. Also present with us is the history of appropriation from the taking of Native people land to the extracting of information from Black and brown bodies in the name of medical advancement. I'd like to take a moment to acknowledge the Ramaytush Ohlone people, who are the traditional custodians of this land. We pay our respects to the Ramaytush Ohlone elders, past, present, and future who call this place the land that UCSF hospitals, research laboratories, and classrooms occupy their home.

I'd also like to take a moment to acknowledge the few individuals who are sacrificed for the advancement of medicine. These include Carter Howard, Frederick Moss, and the Black men who were subjects of the Tuskegee study of untreated syphilis in the "negro male." Also, Elmer Allen, a Black Pullman

Porter living in Richmond, California who, in 1947 had a continuous painful knee. He decided to attend a free clinic ran by UCSF. There, he was injected with plutonium and later had his leg amputated. And Henrietta Lacks, the 30-year-old African American woman whose cells continue to promote our collective immortality.

I'd also like to contribute to our discussion today by not only making this reference that history is present, but the present is also present. It has been almost one year when videos made by witnesses and security cameras of George Floyd's murder became public. While this type of treatment is not new, the footage extended the visibility of police brutality killing Black Americans beyond red line communities and into spaces populated by people who have benefited from residential segregation. As the 1964 movie *Nothing but A Man* brought the lens of a Black man's experience in America's apartheid to viewers, so did the cell phone recordings of George Floyd's murder. Today, as we are turning into this panel discussion, millions of Americans are turning into the trial of one of the police officers charged with this murder. We discuss race and racism and medicine within this context.

And finally, I'd like to suggest that medical research is a social activity that is carried out through a coordinated network of scientists who are influenced by many things including the sociological concept of race. Race as a social construct is a concept that has been molded by racism and the persistent delusion of white supremacy. As Ta-Nehisi Coates reminds us, race is the child of racism, not the father. I'm hoping this framework might help us in making sense of unfair practices in genetic research and healthcare, including the disproportionate data collection practices in genome-wide association studies, which privileges the population of European descent. This type of white framing in research is often operationalized automatically, leaving many stunned when its presence is revealed, often by researchers who are considered outside of the respective scientific fields. Read outsiders in this case as to be sociologists, anthropologists, and historians. So, like most of you joining us today, I'm looking forward to hearing from our panelists and I would like to get started in hearing some of the initial responses from the presentations that we heard from Dr. Ziv and Dr. Hernandez and also to hear a little bit about the video and some of the reactions to that. So, what we've been doing in the past in the other sessions is that we've just been starting by calling upon certain panelists, and I'm gonna do so now in a moderation format. I will start with Dr. Connor.

DENISE CONNOR: Thank you so much and thank you for having me again today. I hope I can offer some perspective coming from medical education in this conversation. I wanted to just echo something that Aimee just discussed, which has to do with the risk of talking about these topics with our learners in a historical way, and the way that we lose credibility, and we break trust with learners when we do that. I love Stephen Richmond's point that teaching comes in all directions, and in many ways our students have been leading the way in these conversations so far. And because of that, because students have had to do their own discovery of the history of racism and medicine and bring that to faculty, there is already a sense of distrust when faculty then want to talk with students about things that are steeped in that history. So, I think a really key lesson that we all need to really think about is when these issues are so tightly linked with sort of real intergenerational trauma, present day trauma, it's our obligation to own up to that racist history when we talk about these things, and that before we can move forward talk about genetics we need to acknowledge where that history is and where that history should be in this conversation. And then, once we do that, I think we can then begin to have conversations about restorative justice and how can we salvage what's good in genetics in an effort to get towards equity and healthcare. So, I just wanted to sort of echo that point.

AIMEE MEDEIROS: Thank you. Dr. Dasgupta?

SHOUMITA DASGUPTA: Thank you again, for including me in this very important conversation. I just wanted to refer back to a very important point emphasized by both Drs. Hernandez and Ziv about the absolute necessity of having diversity in genetic studies in order to be able to reap the benefit of these developments for populations across the world. But, also hearkening back to Dr. Medeiros's comments about history, geneticists have not always done good in this space. One story that we can think about has to do with the Havasupai indigenous peoples hearkening from the deep areas of the Grand Canyon and their agreement with local researchers to be able to study the genetic basis of diabetes in the community, and then those researchers going on to do further studies once they have the DNA in hand, looking at things like the genetic basis of schizophrenia without explicit permission of the tribal members. And this just highlights the absolute necessity of partnering properly with people who are participating in this research. So, there's this saying that's often used, which I think is quite relevant in this context, which is 'not about us without us'. And I think that's a really important concept to think about in this context.

AIMEE MEDEIROS: Thank you. Dr. Rajkovic?

ALEKSANDER RAJKOVIC: Hi. Good morning and I thank you for letting me participate in this. I would like to congratulate Elad, Ryan, and Matt for putting a great population genetics primer that was very, very clear. As a clinical geneticist – I'm not a population genetics – we usually look at mendelian genetics, meaning rare diseases that present either in pediatric populations prenatally or in the adulthood. Usually, American College of Medical Genetics and their guidelines that are currently used to interpret these genetic sequencing is actually relatively population, race, and ethnicity agnostic. However, it does actually influence our ability to interpret even these results because we don't understand the genetic architecture of all the populations across the world. And there have been several situations where a family from Middle East or from Southeastern Asia presents with a disorder and our laboratory says we don't know how to interpret these genetic variants. But clearly, these variants are causing the disease. But because we don't have a good information in our databases of what the genetic variation is, I have to put on my clinical hat and overrule the laboratory and say these variations actually do cause a disease in this individual.

Some groups have embraced genetics very well. We know that a lot of the Ashkenazi Jews have embraced carrier screening and they have really pushed carrier screening in their populations because they're at risk for certain diseases given their population structures. And I think that in many ways, they have used genetics as a way to better the outcomes of their care. Other groups, unfortunately because of the history of racism, do not want to use genetics and approach it with disdain and distrust. And I think that these are the issues in terms of participation in our studies. Increasing diversity are the barriers that we are actually faced as researchers and also as clinicians where we try to use genetics in diverse populations, and especially in populations where history of genetics, explaining inferiority and superiority, utilizing those tools to try to somehow explain socioeconomic and structural racism differences in terms of biology, are actually (unfortunately) backfiring.

This history is backfiring because, as we see, the participation in research especially among minority groups is lagging behind the white populations. In part, this is also due to the lack of infrastructure across the world. I'm happy to see that there are now over 40 countries that are trying to sequence part of the populations for us to better understand the diversity. There is also the Human Heredity and Health Project that is ongoing in Africa, that is run by Africans and enabled by United States and Europe to try to increase diversity and better understanding of African populations, because after all, we all came out of Africa, and we are much less diverse than the African populations are. And so, this is all actually moving in the right direction. But the important problem to maintain is data sharing, because if you're going to use ancestry in our medical records and in refining individual's geography, we need to have access to all the diverse data that is sitting in national or other data banks. And so, these are some of the barriers that will have to be overcome if you're going to fully utilize the studies that are ongoing across the world.

AIMEE MEDEIROS: Thank you so much for those remarks. I'd like to take some of the remarks that we just had and connect them to the presentation through a question. Ancestry is a genetic tool and is a continuous measure, according to Dr. Hernandez. But in the presentations, both speakers created categories of ancestry that seemed to sometimes mean self-reported race and sometimes it meant most dominant genetic ancestry grouping. I'm wondering if there's a way in which we can reconcile this. I'll start with Dr. Hernandez.

RYAN HERNANDEZ: It's a great point. I think that there are some challenges that people perceive when thinking of continuous or quantitative measures such as ancestries. And sometimes, it's just perceived as easier to think about these dichotomous categories in certain types of analyses. When some of us see potential challenges, others of us see opportunity and I think that the decision to think about race and ethnicity as sort of these discrete categories versus ancestry really boils down to the types of questions that you're trying to ask and the ability to integrate people who are able to think about the ways in which we can leverage the information that's contained within the genome, to better use the information than simple dichotomous categories. The use of race and ethnicity has a very fraught history, but as Dr. Ziv has suggested, there is value in using that as a prior mechanism to get people involved in studies that are underrepresented, that have been historically excluded from studies, because we don't have genetic information on everybody and until we do it's hard to access individuals who have been historically excluded from the biomedical research infrastructure without that information. And so, I think that there are ways of bringing in and using all of the information at hand, but it needs a concerted effort to do so.

AIMEE MEDEIROS: Thank you. I'm going to push this a little bit further and I'm going to use some evidence in order for us to be able to discuss this a little bit more specifically. I'm coming to this as a historian – so, coming in this from the outside looking in – and I was curious if we could discuss the second to the last slide of Dr. Ziv's presentation where in which we saw that, on the left-hand column, there was the heading of race/ancestry, where actually, these two terms are combined through the slash. [see Fig. XX] And I'm just curious, how is that, or is that, useful? Or how could this be kind of evidence towards maybe a misunderstanding of some of the discussion? Or also maybe a little bit about how there is concern about the conflating of these terms and how race and ancestry are used interchangeably or are actually being connected through added punctuation in that case.

ELAD ZIV: Yeah, so if I can respond. I think this slide was the table from the NCI website, so I apologize to anyone who didn't like it. And if anyone from the NCI is listening, please fund me. No, just kidding. But I think that you're right. I think that there is some conflation here, and in that case, I'm actually not sure exactly how that table was put together. In some of those studies the genetic information is available, and you can actually subset it even more; I think it wasn't available perhaps to all the people putting that table together. But I guess I would say, once we get the genetic information, once we get the data, it's actually relatively easy. But I think the point I was trying to make with taking that slide is that it was at least five to one, if not ten to one, for some groups, and even worse for other groups that if you're doing sort of a ten to one data bias, you can't even start making conclusions. And I think the point of that slide is just to sort of like ... how did we get here, and to start the conversation really, how do we undo that?

And I think that one of the ways perhaps to undo that is to recognize that it's a problem and to recruit and, as far as I can tell, you need to recruit based on self-identification even for the purpose of enhancing ancestry because we don't really have an ability to infer anyone's ancestry without genotyping them. We can't genotype them until we recruit them. I think there's a problem of recruitment. It's a problem that kind of has been built for decades. It wasn't like somebody went out and tried to do this ten to one or five to one sort of bias. I think it was just sort of people had like here are the studies we have let's run the arrays, let's find the most genes. But I think it was the kind of the structural racism that existed in genetic studies for decades, came home to roost with the introduction of genomic association studies. So, I'll stop there.

AIMEE MEDEIROS: Okay, let's hear from Dr. Connor and then Dr. Dasgupta.

DENISE CONNOR: Thanks so much. I wanted to just add one thing. I think certainly what we're saying – and I agree with – is that the problem becomes when we are very reductionist, and we want to use a small number of discrete categories to describe what is clearly a continuum. But then the conflict of how do we get that continuum, that information.

But I actually wanted to take a minute to talk about the patient here. I've heard a lot about the problem and the barrier being that individuals don't know their ancestry, and that therefore we need to use socio-political character, their race, instead. While it may be true that people don't know their ancestry, I think when we talk, we talk with our patients about ancestry as separate from their race, we can really create opportunities for personal narrative and individuation that are really important for patients. So, giving people a chance to reflect on the impact of the diaspora on the loss of their family's knowledge about distant ancestry, for example, could be a very healing thing to do in the healthcare setting and could help us to avoid stereotyping and bias by getting to know our patients' unique family histories, what they know and what they don't know, and why they know things and why they don't know things. Sitting with our patients to learn about that, I think, could be very empowering for patients. Even though we don't yet have all the information we need to have to make clinical decisions once we know that ancestry, I actually think talking to patients about ancestry as separate from race would be quite empowering.

SHOUMITA DASGUPTA: If I may add on to the wonderful comments from Drs. Ziv and Connor – I was also thinking about the impact on the individual patients and thinking about the question of, why are we using race and ancestry in the clinical context. The real reason is that we don't have the actual risk factors identified in many cases. Is the risk factor for the disease racism? Is the risk factor exposure to environmental toxins? Or is it that variant at position 2694 on chromosome 5? What is it actually that is causing this increased risk that is observed in various human populations? And so, race or ancestry, whichever flavor is being used in the context of clinical care, is used as a placeholder until we have better information. And so, we're really in that in between liminal space where we're trying to identify the true risk factors so that we can make more precise predictions about an individual's risk.

The other thing I would point out is, when we think about an individual's identity and how it's actually documented in somebody's medical record, what we need to realize is that there's so many different ways this information is documented. Sometimes, it is self-reported. Sometimes, you're only allowed to check one box, so you're not allowed to be admixed actually in certain record forms. Sometimes, it's based on just being eyeballed on your way into the clinic. So, really there's just such a range in which this information actually enters the medical record and therefore clinical diagnostic reasoning.

AIMEE MEDEIROS: Thank you. Let's hear from Dr. Rajkovic and then Dr. Hernandez.

ALEKSANDER RAJKOVIC: Yeah, I do want to reiterate the fact that holistically looking at the patient and especially the family pedigree is an extremely important tool which unfortunately is not easy to do in a clinical setting where you have 10-15 minutes per patient. But I would argue that family pedigree can give you so much information about the background of the individual that is so unique about that particular individual. And then you can hopefully then personalize your care based on that. As well, it's important any variant that you may identify that may have clinical significance needs to be put in the context of the family, because it may have significantly different meanings in different families both in terms of penetrance and how it's going to manifest. So, again, I agree.

A lot of what we do is reductionist, but we always have to pull ourselves out of that and we need to use many tools before we actually label something as significant or not significant. And that's where experience and the clinical acumen comes into regular clinical care. So, I think from that perspective, that is an important piece that needs to be held to account because I still had ... many of our rounds where we get stuck trying to interpret one variant and how it may cause this or that. And again, those kinds of approaches have also been used to justify certain physical traits, to justify certain intellectual traits which have been debunked by many studies. That such reductionism is a total mismeasure of an individual, both clinically and otherwise.

AIMEE MEDEIROS: Dr. Hernandez and then Dr. Ziv.

RYAN HERNANDEZ: I really appreciate the comments from Drs. Connor and Dasgupta. I think that it's critical to think about what the driving factors are and whether race and ethnicity means something in a biological context in the context of these studies that we're doing if it's actually necessary to use as a filter or as a mechanism for recruiting individuals with diverse ancestry. And these are things that we need to study very deeply and think about very, very seriously.

One of the interesting components of thinking about ancestry is that, because it's something that we can't necessarily assess just by looking at ourselves in the mirror, surprises can pop up and people can identify, can learn they have more or less ancestry than they might have expected or hoped. And there can be a certain amount of stigma in that as well. Growing up as a Latino – my father's Mexican American, my mother's white – I always found myself too much of a Latino to fit in with my white friends, and too white to fit in with my Latino friends. This is something that I can tell just from looking at me, and then it was sort of verified when I did my genetic ancestry analysis and see that I have 20% Amerindigenous ancestry. What does that mean? How do I feel about myself? How do I check those boxes? Do I check the white box? Do I check other? Do I check mixed?

I have almost 4% African ancestry. What do I do with that information? These things, as a population geneticist, I finally have some sense of how I would use that information, but not until recently. This is not a concept that's very easy to disseminate and to have a concrete discussion with people about, unless you have a large number of trained individuals who are capable of thinking about this. And I would love to see that be the case. I would love to have outreach in this regard, to increase representation from people across the spectrum of humanity. I really love the quote that Dr. Dasgupta used, 'not about us without us.' I think that really captures exactly what we need to do and why we need to spend so much effort diversifying the biomedical research workforce in order to make sure that these concepts are adequately addressed and included when we're designing these studies and when we're actually moving forward with how we handle clinical care.

AIMEE MEDEIROS: Dr. Ziv?

ELAD ZIV: Yeah, thank you. I guess I wanted to also reflect on something Dr. Connor said about the personal history of individuals, and actually also what Dr. Rajkovic said about the history of families. I found it really instructive later in my career, or I guess the middle of my career, to start going to the genetic counseling, they tumor genetics board where they talk about families in the context of mutations. They get, actually, a lot of history, a lot more history than we usually get in clinical medicine about origin of families from very precise regions of the globe, at least to the degree that people know. And the people know a fair amount more than, I think, perhaps we give them credit for, which I think is what Connor was saying. And the reason they do that is not just because they're curious and interested. They actually learn a fair amount more about the individual mutations that they are seeking to understand. And particularly, because they're dealing with very rare mutations, those tend to cluster in very much smaller genetic pools.

And so, I think that goes back into the question of categorization and why is it useful and what point is it useful for in the genetic arena. I think from the perspective of the genetics work, if you're thinking about a particular variant, a really rare variant, then probably race is going to be far too coarse of a tool to use for even for recruitment. And having a lot more information about more proximal geographic origins or more precise geographic origins is probably more useful. So, I think we really need to be careful about why we're using it and how we're thinking about recruiting.

But I guess I want to reflect back to Dr. Medeiros earlier questions, what potential benefits there are of using race. I think this was raised in the introductory video. So, one example of a disease that's been studied in terms of disparities is prostate cancer. I think many of the clinicians and epidemiologists who are listening are probably aware that prostate cancer incidence is higher in Black men in the United States in comparison to Blacks in whites and lower in comparison to both of those groups in Asians. And knowing that information, certain researchers actually recruited African Americans into their studies – Black men into their studies – with precisely the question of whether they could find genetic variants to help understand this difference. And they have found some, and there's a sort of a long list of papers that have been published. And this doesn't explain everything. It certainly doesn't explain disparities that arise from treatment, from referral, from screening, and so on. So, there's a lot of other biases that occur that are completely independent of the genetics. But the difference in incidence at least, can be potentially attributed to a very small number of variants that are only present in a very small number of individuals on average. So, in that case, race is not useful in the clinical space ultimately. It's not really race that's the driver of the disease at all. But if the researcher thinks about it and can do the proper studies, then in my mind at least, that's potentially beneficial to the people who potentially carry that variant and then ultimately hopefully can be screened if the genetic information gets back to them.

AIMEE MEDEIROS: I'd like to ask a question about this. I think it relates back to the previous discussion that we were having earlier today. I hear what you're saying, but at the same time, if we continue to use race as the deciphering element that is going to construct this study, does it not perpetuate the belief that race is a biological construct which is very dangerous given the fact that race is not only a social construct but one that has been molded by racism and white supremacy? And so, if we continue to use race as this framework, we miss – and this has been referenced in the Q&A throughout this morning – we miss some of the social determinants of health, structural forces of health like racism, other elements that are really having a huge impact that continue to get left out of framing studies because we fall back on race, which is problematic and actually harmful.

ALEKSANDER RAJKOVIC: I mean, I think that what is going on is the fact that if you don't try to seek out diverse groups of populations in your study, you will end up primarily with white populations participating. And so how does one actually increase and diversify their population base? And NIH currently requires us to recruit patients based on various racial groups that have been accepted by the government and so on. And so, everybody tries to bin people into these groups to satisfy the NIH requirements and get that grant funded. What is important is not to use race as a variable to somehow stratify people between white and non-white individuals. That's when you get into troubles. That's when a lot of the studies end up finding associations which may be spurious or non-biological. But I think race in itself, if you actually just recruit by race, every group, white, Black, Hispanic, is highly diverse. Very, very diverse. And so then, the question for investigators how do we capture that diversity separate from the binning that we currently are obliged to do for NIH applications? And that's what a challenge becomes. How do you actually take those individuals and really use them as diverse populations instead of looking at them just as five different populations?

AIMEE MEDEIROS: Dr. Ziv? And then we're going to turn it to an audience question.

ELAD ZIV: Yeah, I guess some of the trouble I have with the 'race is or is not biology' makes it sort of dichotomous. So, if you mean 'it is biology', what are you saying? Or if you're saying, 'it's not biology', what are you saying? I think we've all agreed – or I'll just say – I agree with the idea that race is a social construct and that, as outlined by many speakers, it was created at a certain time. I think where perhaps some disagreements arise is what information race is capturing about ancestry and to what degree does that capture information about genotype. And my argument would be that race does capture information about ancestry, albeit imperfectly. And we know to some degree where it misses things or where it really messes up.

Dr. Hernandez talked about admixed populations and there are lots of examples where it's a very imprecise tool, particularly when it's collected in a categorical way. There are ways to collect information about race where you can say – and I think increasingly studies are doing that – saying 'check all that apply.' You can ask questions about people, not just themselves but about their parents and so on. But I guess to me it seems like where we say, well since race is a social construct that, therefore, cannot offer any information about ancestry or genotype, and therefore it is inherently scientifically flawed and fraught problematically to think of it in that domain. I can see the fact that you're saying linking it creates problems and I acknowledge that, and I think that that's a really important thing to carry with us in our minds.

I guess the counter to that is the concern I have is it cuts both ways in the sense that if we end up trying to completely remove it from the arena when we do genetic studies, we end up with biases that then create new disparities that I don't think were intentional but end up hurting people. I feel like it's a difficult and fraught discussion. I guess that's why we're all here. But I think it's really being back to the title as sort of race conscious sort of thinking about it, why are we using it? Have we really thought about it from the perspective of the sociologist as well as the patient when we when we use it in the genetic arena?

AIMEE MEDEIROS: Thank you. I am now going to turn it to Dr. Dehlendorf, who will be offering us a question from the audience.

CHRISTINE DEHLENDORF: Thank you, Dr. Medeiros. This is a related question to the last comments by Dr. Ziv, which is how can and should genetic researchers and those using genetic technologies in the clinical space engage with the history of genetics including eugenics to both build trust and avoid reproducing oppression?

SHOUMITA DASGUPTA: I think these things need to be discussed in training as people are going through their advanced training to become clinicians or to become investigators. Some folks are not aware of these historical examples and maybe aren't aware of the population genetic variation that describes within group or between group variation. So, this is a subject – I think Dr. Medeiros referred about insiders and outsiders in the past – and I think we really need to talk about interdisciplinary education and exploring these topics across the spectrum of expertise.

I'll just put a plug out there. I did compile some resources, an anti-racism toolkit for genetics educators that I'll ask the organizers to put into the chat in case folks want to refer to those resources. And we're also starting a national initiative through the APHMG, the Association of Professors of Human and Medical Genetics, to work with educators that have already demonstrated a curriculum that actually disentangles the understanding of race and can actually help people to shed racist ideas that they might walk into a classroom with just based on life experience. And so, this particular curriculum has been demonstrated as being effective in the high school space, and we're looking at adapting it into medical school and other spaces where people are talking about genetics. So, for folks who are interested in that, please feel free to reach out to me or to just visit aphmg.org to see our upcoming workshop.

AIMEE MEDEIROS: Thank you. Dr. Connor?

DENISE CONNOR: I appreciate that comment a lot. I'm looking forward to looking at that resource. I was going to just add as a broad comment – as some students have done for faculty, we want to encourage all of our learners to really come at this with a critical mindset because ultimately, we want to graduate folks who can recognize and unpack racism in medicine and disrupt the insidious impact it has for our patients and community members. And I think that means really not teaching dogmatically and teaching in a way that encourages question asking. Kevin Kumashiro, who has written a lot about anti-oppressive education, has some wonderful examples of the kinds of questions we should be asking or getting our students to habitually ask.

So, for example, one question I love that he has is 'just as we're more open to learning only certain things, how might many in science communities be more open to addressing only certain issues, asking only certain questions, using only certain methods or communicating only certain findings?' And I think it comes back to what Dr. Grubbs said, which is this obsession we have with race and the fact that it keeps coming up again and again says something about our history in medicine and our current way of thinking about race. And so, how can we really engage with students as co-learners in understanding these things and really having open discussions about these issues?

ELAD ZIV: I'm not sure this addresses this precise question, but I think that what has come up here is to really be very careful. I mean, I've advocated for the use of race as a tool for recruitment, racial identification as a tool for recruitment to enhance genetic ancestry. But I really think there has been a lot written about the misuse of race to infer associations about biology without evidence. I think that's where we still fail in current biomedical research. And I think that, in the clinical research community, we need to be really careful and really thoughtful if we put race in the model, why did we do that? If we report it, why are we reporting it? And be exceptionally careful about that. And as Dr. Medeiros called out the slide that I used, to really be careful about when we're using ancestry not to conflate it with race or vice versa. I think that maybe good research practices will help engender more trust in the future. We can't undo the past, but I think we could try and be as scrupulous as we possibly can about the present.

ALEKSANDER RAJKOVIC: I'm a strong believer that we know that individual differences are greater than intercontinental differences in many cases, and that really, the goal of personalized and precision medicine is to apply our knowledge to that individual and not to spread it across the group because group contains individuals that are quite diverse in who they are, what they are, and what their capabilities are. And so, really, how do we get to the goal because of course, a lot of us as epidemiologists – I'm not going to count myself as an epidemiologist although I have been in many of those studies – is that we try to average everyone, treat everyone as one widget and try to then apply those methodologies on the masses.

But the challenge is, how do you apply to N=1? And that has been very, very difficult to do. And when you do that, then the race is gone. I mean, I'm talking from biological purposes. Of course, I'm not talking about a sociocultural and other political issue that the race will persist and affect the healthcare. But in terms of your biological propensity to disorders, your genetics will only give you a predisposition. What is your predisposition to something? And how do we apply to N=1 instead of grouping it into these very imprecise bins is, I think, a challenge.

CHRISTINE DEHLENDORF: This leads us to the final question, and it's definitely inspired by some of the discussions that we had in preparation for this panel today. We've been talking a little bit behind the scenes about what could we forecast, what this discussion could look like in five years or the use of race in clinical practice or the use of ancestry in clinical practice in five years. Will this discussion be seen as something that was specific of a certain time or do you predict that the use of race in which how we're using it today will continue, whether it's with the recruitment of subjects for studies or in clinical practice. And so, I'm going to open up to the panelists and see if you'd like to do a little bit of prediction here and we'll wage bets, too.

RYAN HERNANDEZ: I'm not much of a betting man usually, so I won't wager much, but my hope is that with precision medicine, we move to an era where we aren't comparing individuals to some perceived population that they might belong to, whether it be by ancestry or by race or ethnicity at all, but we compare those individuals to themselves, where we have an understanding of what an individual's normal is throughout their life and we can see when things deviate from the expectation for that individual. That is the goal, in my mind, and trying to compare to race/ethnicity or ancestry is actually just a stop gap measure in order and until we can find a better way to access what an individual pattern should be.

AIMEE MEDEIROS: And do you think we'll be there by 2026?

RYAN HERNANDEZ: There should be nothing holding us back. Anything that's holding us back will, if we're not there by that point, we will have failed.

AIMEE MEDEIROS: Got it. Dr. Dasgupta?

SHOUMITA DASGUPTA: Thank you. I was going to comment that, as we consider the future, one important fact to remember is that our populations are becoming more and more mixed in terms of ancestry. So, these individual designations by race are becoming less and less meaningful. They weren't great to begin with and they're getting worse. And so, we are getting to that point, as Dr. Rejkovic was talking about, where we need to really be thinking about the individual, what their risk factors are, and Dr. Hernandez was talking about. The work that's ongoing right now to develop an understanding of what those risk factors are. We're moving towards the future where genomic analysis of individuals is going to be more and more routine, and we see that already with studies that are looking at newborn genomic sequencing and using that as a prediction. I don't think we're going to be there in 2026, but I think that is the direction we're going in the long run.

AIMEE MEDEIROS: Dr. Rajkovic and then Dr. Ziv. You are on mute. We cannot hear you.

ALEKSANDER RAJKOVIC: Just to support the move towards more individualization of precision medicine. We now know that therapeutics are actually now being developed toward specific variants. Also, CAR-T therapies are developed, very personalized to your tumor. So, I think we are moving in that direction. My prediction is that ancestry will be used more to see whether it can improve clinical care, so I think we're going to have probably some studies over the next five years using ancestry more as an assay tool. I still think that race, because it's embedded because of the historical, cultural, social, and legal processes – will remain at the societal level, and I think that unfortunately, will always color what physicians do, because we do not work in a vacuum. Now, could our efforts lead to deconstruction of these issues? I would like to be optimistic, but the reality is that we're just a very small part of what happens in the society, and unfortunately physicians have always been influenced by what happens in the societal level, how they interpret things and embed them. But I hope that at the government level, these movements also change and move away from using race in our politics and in our other discourses, because I think that also can color what we do with our patients, too.

AIMEE MEDEIROS: Dr. Ziv and then Dr. Connor.

ELAD ZIV: Yeah, so I think I want to also echo the concept of more individualization. I guess I want to make a comment about ancestry. I think ancestry is sort of also a proxy and kind of like a short-term deal. I think it'll be perhaps useful in the next a few years – maybe two to five or something – and then hopefully after that, it becomes less useful as we've learned a lot more about genetics of all of the whole world. Maybe five is probably over ambitious, but once we learn enough about the genetics of the whole world, then we actually can from the genetics perspective go to genotype. So, I think it'll be more individualized. I think actually, there's a wonderful paper by Dr. Hernandez about low frequency variants – really, really private variants – that we share just probably with our immediate family members, that actually drive a lot of the heritability that we're all ultimately interested in. I personally believe those will be really important and ultimately, if we can get the information from them from the genetics perspective, help all of our patients a lot more. And so, I guess I think I think ancestry's got a maybe two-to-seven-year kind of window of being useful. I think that hopefully after that, the genetics becomes a lot more useful and interesting. I think race stays because it's a much more complex, rich, and as we have discussed, problematic, variable, or I guess framework. But still, will capture a lot more about how we're practicing. I'll just say, in my clinical domain we look at, in our clinic, how we're doing in terms of managing vaccinations or screening and so on by race, and that's really all are we giving equitable care. So, I still think we hopefully will and should use it from that perspective. And we'll stop there.

AIMEE MEDEIROS: So, it sounds like ancestry will be the Blackberry of genetics research in about five years. Dr. Connor?

DENISE CONNOR: I appreciate all the comments. I think the only thing I was going to also add is, precision medicine is exciting. It's exciting to imagine thinking about people as individuals, for sure, and moving beyond a lot of the problems that come with grouping people into these actually very diverse groups that have social and political origins. But I also just want to remind us that genetics is, of course, just one small part of disease, and we need we have issues with housing, how people are dealt with, the social justice system, these huge impacts on health that need funding and actually may have benefits that outweigh spending as much resource on precision medicine as on these other social factors and structural factors of health. And so, trying to find the right balance for that in the next five years I think is important, because we have so many needs in our society that have to do with racism and structural racism that I would like to see our energy and funds going towards. Not to discount the importance of precision medicine, but how do we balance those things? I do think that's an important conversation to be having.

AIMEE MEDEIROS: Thank you so much. That's a wonderful way to wrap up this panel. I appreciate and honor all of you.

KIRSTEN BIBBINS-DOMINGO: Let me add my thanks to all of the panelists and to Dr. Medeiros for moderating it so well. I really appreciate all of you and your contributions to this discussion. Let me just say that this wraps up the first three parts of our series. We began with history, and we have ended most of our panel discussions looking forward to the future. But, as our historian Dr. Medeiros reminds us, history is our present. And so, I think our challenge is to actually wrestle with many of the hard questions that we asked our speakers but also that we are all faced with and trying to think about how to apply their perspectives to our work ensuring that we are at an anti-racist institution and that we are doing the best for our patients and that we are providing the best possible care to all of our patients in the most equitable manner possible.

And so, I think that, as Dr. Fernandez said in our very first session, this is going to be hard work. But we are we are up to the challenge of doing this work as Dr. Grubbs reminds us, and I hope as many of you as possible will be able to engage with the ongoing discussions on this topic. Again, if you are interested in both reflecting with others on what you've heard during these sessions as well as offering us an opportunity to apply this in a way that we can make our teaching, our research, and our practice better across our UC medical campuses, please join at one of these discussions. We really need people to register ahead of time and you'll see that the two on medical education and research are taking place in two weeks from today, on Wednesday, and the clinical practice session in three weeks from today. These are all Wednesday morning sessions. Please join. This will be the opportunity to have more small group discussions on this very important topic. And again then, just in closing, let me thank all of our speakers, our steering committee, our students, everyone who has really participated in how we have tried to construct this conversation, and look forward to this being just the first of many more conversations on this important topic. Thank you so much.

Introductory Remarks

KIRSTEN BIBBINS-DOMINGO: Good morning everyone. Welcome to the last of our sessions on *Racism and Race: The Use of Race and Medicine and Implications for Health Equity*. My name is Kirsten Bibbins-Domingo. I am the Vice Dean for Population Health and Health Equity in the UCSF School of Medicine and Chair of the Department of Epidemiology and Biostatistics here. I appreciate all of you who are joining us.

So just to remind you about the series that we embarked upon at the end of March. We have been focused over a number of weeks on exploring the use of race and racial categorizations in medicine and the implications for health equity. We started on March 24th, laying the foundation by exploring historical context and current perspectives on this issue. These have been Wednesday morning half day sessions and they're all available on video through our website. We then moved from the historical context to a series of three case studies to delve deeper into how we use racial categories in medicine, how we use them in the context of prescribing medications, how we use them in diagnostic algorithms like the glomerular filtration rate (GFR), and how we use them in polygenic risk scores.

In all of these conversations, we've been trying to explore what we might do differently in our education, clinical care, and research missions. We want to apply an understanding of both the historical context and its application in these particular contexts, representing all of the many ways that we continue to use racial categories. We then had a great set of discussions over a two-day period where we focused on our three mission areas. We invited conversation with many of you across our UC Medical Center campuses who are dedicated to our teaching, clinical care, and research missions to try to think of the application of the earlier presentations to these mission areas. Our goal now is to think about the synthesis and next steps.

We have the synthesis from the three discussion sessions that will form the basis for our panel discussion today. The written syntheses of these are available on open proposals, and our intent of putting them on open proposals is to invite you to comment on these, because our hope is that this conversation extends to more concrete action steps, and to do that we want to engage as many of you in this conversation as possible. There's also a library of resources on our web page that many of the speakers in the earlier sessions provided.

Our collective vision is to implement an anti-racist approach to how we use racial categorizations in medicine, and our goals for today are to explore with several of the leaders on our campuses who participated in these discussions what we've learned and how we hope to activate next steps. Again, a reminder of our shared values: differences of opinion are expected and welcome. As you know, we've had a range of opinions expressed throughout these sessions, and that is what we want. We want to have the more nuanced conversations, to not shy away from disagreements, but we always want to do this with respect for speakers and discussants, because our goal is to collectively move forward in the best way possible.

I am really thrilled today to invite a great group of people to discuss this topic. Throughout, we've had incredible faculty who have both helped us in planning as a part of our steering committee, helped us in leading the discussions, and helped us as speakers and panelists for prior sessions. I really appreciate my colleagues here who will help us to understand more about the in-depth discussions. These are a Dr. Denise Connor from UCSF, Dr. Hal Collard from UCSF, Dr. Takesha Cooper from UC Riverside, Dr. Kevin Grumbach from UCSF, Dr. Helena Hansen from UCLA, Dr. Malcolm John from UCSF, and Dr. Catherine Lucey from UCSF. I've asked these individuals who are leaders on their campuses in these mission areas to help us to understand the nature of the conversations that we had in these smaller groups, and to help us think through our next steps forward. We were really fortunate to have participants from all of our UC medical school campuses and from our different mission areas participate. Our goal here is to engage as many of you as possible in these discussions because the answers are not always exactly clear of what the next step forward is and I think we can arrive at clarity on the next step forward, because we do have to make some steps forward by doing this together. So thank you to the panelists for joining us today, and to all of you who have participated in these discussions.

Moderated Discussion

KIRSTEN BIBBINS-DOMINGO: I want to begin by asking you to reflect, from your domains of clinical, research, and education, what were the things that were most impactful for you either in the earlier presentations that we had or in the discussions where you could talk with your colleagues about the education mission for example? And I'm going to start with education. I know that that Catherine and Takesha participated there, and maybe others of you did as well. I'd invite you to reflect on what you thought were most impactful in those conversations. Catherine?

CATHERINE LUCEY: Thanks, Kirsten. It's really been a pleasure to participate in this. I think, like most people who engaged, we all learned a great deal and benefited from some very spirited and thoughtful conversations with our colleagues across the UC system. So I appreciate your bringing us all together.

I think from an educational perspective, there were several lessons that came out as we listened and also as we worked on the last seminar. The first is that everyone who has participated agrees that some form of transformation in medical education environment is necessary as a key strategy to unravel the consequences and manifestations of structural racism in our health and health care systems, in our biomedical research systems, and in our educational system. So, there was I think universal agreement for that.

I think there were a lot of insights that I want to just touch upon that really speak to scale and scope of issues that I think merit deep discussion and strategic intervention on. The first is that when you think about medical education you often think about content, but that is just the beginning of the work that we need to do. And content in terms of teaching about these issues of race and racism and also controversies, nuances, and disagreements has to begin with embedding this in the history, sociology, and psychology of structural racism and the way it manifests in how we teach, who we teach, who teaches, and how we engage with our patients.

It's insufficient just to add a recognition of unconscious bias or how to deal with microaggressions. That's the tip of the iceberg and if it's context-free without an understanding of the systems in which we work and how they've been constructed to systemically disadvantaged populations, I think we will fail. It will be sort of a tree without roots, in essence. But it also has to recognize that curricular content is not the only way that racism or race might be adversely dealt with in the medical education environment. We have to think about redesigning all aspects of our educational environment, which includes how we assess, evaluate, counsel, promote, recommend careers, and support all of our learners particularly those coming from groups traditionally excluded by medicine.

I think the other thing that we talked a lot about is that with our institutions, the scale and scope is substantial. When you say medical education, there's this instant reaction that we should just change the way we educate medical students and then eventually they'll change our institutions. But that's a 10-to-15-year process and we can't wait that long. We have people who are dying today because of health care disparities and health disparities, and whose careers are impacted because of educational disparities and discrimination. So we need simultaneously an educational strategy that tackles people in all parts of the medical education ecosystem: that's students, residents, faculty, and health professionals, and that addresses the systems and structures that surround those people in our institution so that we can make sure that we can accelerate the embrace of anti-racism competencies and don't dilute interventions towards anti-racism by then throwing those medical students into environments that are not anti-racist.

I think the other point I wanted to make is that we have to accept that this work will continue if not forever then for the foreseeable future. This is a complex problem. We will never be finished with interventions. We will only be ahead of the curve and the interventions that we choose. And we also have to accept that the work can't stop at the borders of our institutions. It really has to go beyond our own individual institutions across the nation for a couple of reasons. The physician workforce is very mobile. We are going to continuously have people coming into our institution who have been educated at, or had careers at, institutions that haven't actually taken this journey. So, we'll need to always have a way of embracing them as new colleagues and also helping them understand how we are viewing these issues and how we expect them to participate in this transformation.

And our learners are impacted by systems that span institutions: the national residency matching program, licensing exams, board certification exams, things like that. And so those also need to be changed to be not to be anti-racist. I think UCSF has a great opportunity, along with our colleagues in the other UC systems, to address these issues and push for national change with the platforms that we have as one of the leading, if not the leading, public institution in the world. And so I think a really important aspect of our work is how we influence things outside of the UC system and work for change that happens more impactfully across the nation.

I'll just close in saying that what's been very clear over the past year is that COVID showed us what was possible when we felt we had no choice but to change because people were dying. I think we have to tap into that same urgency to engage in this transformation because people are still dying of consequences of structural racism. It's just that they die much more quietly without those big headlines in the *New York Times* or on CNN. So, we have to recognize that, without intervention, we will not be serving our patients and our students well. So, with that I'll stop and turn it over to Takesha for her insights. She's been a tremendous contributor in all of the engagements that we've had in this work.

TAKESHA COOPER: Thank you, Catherine. It's difficult to follow you, but I will just point out a couple of things that were meaningful for me, and I'm so grateful to have been able to participate in this series, which I think was excellent.

Early in the series the question was raised, where is racism in all of this? And I think it's important that we continue to acknowledge the role of racism that was embedded in our medical forefathers and really think intentionally and critically about how racism continues to play a role in the outcomes of our patients, in our research design, and how we make clinical decisions, etc. As a training director myself now, the events of the past year have been noticeably exhausting for my residents, for other trainees, and for our students, particularly those trainees of color. And I've had a lot of allies wanting to know what can they do, looking deeper into themselves about how they can contribute to anti-racism, wanting to do the work of learning and reading which has been wonderful to see. And I realized that at my institution, the vast majority of students and trainees are very eager to have these conversations, to do the work, and we need to create the space for them to have the conversation and to tolerate the discomfort that often comes along with these types of conversations. And not just with trainees, but I think faculty need to press themselves to have these conversations with each other, with their trainees as well.

And I'll just close by amplifying Catherine's point that this work really must continue. One of my concerns is that after George Floyd's murder, there was lots of – and it was very surprising to me because I feel like this has been going on for quite some time – there's suddenly a lot of engagement and acknowledgement of a lot of things that have been chronic. And so the concern is, is it going to die down? Is the interest going to wane? Are people going to go back to their regular lives? And I think we have to be very intentional to make sure that doesn't happen that people remain engaged that we continue to work on a day-to-day basis of anti-racism.

KIRSTEN BIBBINS-DOMINGO: Thank you very much, Catherine and Takesha. And let me first just say that our road map for today is for each of the representatives from each of the domains to share their reflections, but then to have more crosstalk across these because one of the things that I think is really highlighted in both Catherine and Takesha's comments is how important, foundational, and urgent it is to address some of these issues within our educational environments. But doing that just in those environments is not going to be helpful because we send our students to do clinical care, to do research, to read and understand the literature, and to other institutions. And part of what I hope today is a little bit more talk across our domain so that we can, even though we'll be doing this work for our lifetime, start doing them across multiple sectors in which we work within our institutions. So thank you for getting us started. I want to invite Hal Collard and Helena Hansen to reflect a little bit from the research perspective. What reflections did you have on this series or in your discussions with your other colleagues who are leading or conducting research across your campuses? Hal and Helena?

HAL COLLARD: Yeah, thanks Kirsten. I have a few comments. First, thank you Kirsten, for involving me in organizing and moderating the clinical and translational research part of this series. It's been great to partner with and learn from listening to you. Congratulations on this session, to you, Stephanie, Christine, the rest of the group. I've learned a tremendous amount listening to and participating in the series. I think we all have.

Catherine mentioned, most fundamentally in my mind, that race as a social construct exists because of racism and that it's complex in how it interacts and relates to research in the pursuit of knowledge. Honestly, the thing that struck me the most, Kirsten, in these sessions is how little thought is given to this issue in a lot of clinical and translational research, and by a lot of clinical and translational researchers. And that needs to change. I think this session really created the space to reflect on, talk about, and educate, and so I've been really appreciative of that.

I want to give you a specific example, and the group a specific example from my own field. I study a condition called idiopathic pulmonary fibrosis. It's a chronic deadly scarring lung disease, and I was taught as a clinical fellow in the early 2000s that it was uncommon in African Americans, in Black populations, a belief that was reinforced by the demographics and cohorts, from tertiary centers like ours, and what has since been refuted in better community-based studies. But this belief, I am sure, has contributed to, and still contributes to, under-diagnosis and delayed diagnosis by me and my colleagues in this space. This has never been meaningfully discussed in our research community, that I'm aware of.

Another example, in the last decade, again in this disease: there's been an explosion of literature in the genetic basis for this. There have been mutations identified in telomerase proteins, polymorphisms in MUC5B, which is a mucin. I went through the literature last night. No one has meaningfully looked the relationship of these genetic abnormalities to race. No one has done that. So why is this? The intersection of genetics and race is complicated. I learned that. I get that from this series. But I'm not sure anyone's even tried to explore that in our literature, so I just wanted to share that with you as a personal reflection on how this series is important to the clinical and translation research community in making us think about the issues of race and racism and how they interact with our research and that we need to attend to them.

In our session on clinical and translational research, we had a number of breakout groups. Maybe all of you did this type of structure. Those breakout groups generated recommendations for next steps or just areas for consideration for our institutions and for our communities. This was a wonderful process and I'm really appreciative of all the energy people put into that. Many of these focused on education and accountability. I think recognizing that some of the work we need to do is just to have this conversation take place. So, for example, developing a mechanism for researchers to obtain consultation related to incorporating race and racism into their research and perhaps tying funding opportunities to use of this service. There are some resources for this, but they're not well appreciated and they're maybe not as well publicized and incentivized, and so I think we as an institution need to think about ways in which we promote that.

Another example: expecting researchers to explicitly name race and racism as important variables or factors in the design, conduct, and interpretation of research projects. How can we as institutions and institutional leaders promote that? Another: developing and requiring training or competencies in the use of race in clinical and translational research. I think this is something that maybe speaks to our later conversation about how we work together, a common ontology or framework for how we even talk about this issue and think about it conceptually.

So maybe in closing, I'll just say I'm committed to working with all of you on this call and the larger community in implementing the recommendations that came up with the goal of elevating race and racism to more central place in our conversation about clinical and translational research. So that's what I took away, Kirsten, most directly.

HELENA HANSEN: Thank you, Hal. I couldn't agree more with what you just said. What I'm really hearing based on the examples you provided from your own research and the examples that you gave of how we could be conducting research differently, you're really calling for the need for a new paradigm. A new paradigm that is biosocial, that integrates bench science, life sciences, as well as clinical research with social, very well informed and nuanced understandings of social processes like racism that are responsible for the inequalities that we see.

I also want to amplify what Catherine Lucey and Takesha Cooper brought up, that a transformation is necessary in education, and I think the same transformation is equally applicable to research. We need to embed it in history, sociology, psychology, perhaps anthropology of structural racism. And we need to, as a part of that, also engage with communities. Because one thing I heard was the need to not stop at the border of the medical school itself. That includes reaching out not only to practitioners outside of academic medicine, but also members of communities directly affected by the inequalities that we're studying.

And so, just briefly, I want to explain. I'm an addiction psychiatrist. I'm also a cultural anthropologist. One thing that is a guiding principle of social science of medicine, and of critical studies of race, that is of the master narrative, the idea that science (including biomedical science and a lot of other aspects of our society) have a story or logic which organizes them. So, an organizing logic or story or narrative of our institutions including biomedicine and that that narrative that master narrative involves a selective perception of reality that confirms the reality, so it leads to self-fulfilling predictions and received wisdom about, for example, the causes of health inequalities that are resistant to change. And I think it's that master narrative that we have to hone in on.

So in academic medicine, there's a very strong master narrative that is individually focused and it includes excellence through individual competition. This applies to scientists and how they make it in their fields. It includes better living through new technologies that in our society are designed for individual consumption, for profit. There's a very strong logic of individual patients and individual scientists who develop consumable products. And these logics imply that health outcomes are driven by individual risk factors and behaviors. So we have scientific disciplines that heavily focus on the individual in order to try to explain racial inequalities in health. And in the world of science, biomedical research, these logics of the individual traits or merits explaining the outcomes and what we see in front of us, including inequalities in who's represented among the scientific workforce.

These narratives imply that Black biomedical scientists, who only receive one to two percent of the NIH R01 grants right now as PIs, that implies that this is because there's a shortage of qualified and motivated individual Black scientists. So I want to bring the institution of biomedical science into this conversation. When pipeline programs increase the number of Black people training in medical science, when those fail to raise the percentage of black NIH-funded PIs, then the unspoken master narrative is that Black people are deficient in the qualities that make excellent scientists. This enables the continuation of a system which, conscious or not, white scientists trained in a select number of individually focused disciplines dominate NIH portfolios, and they continue to positively review and promote, from their own ranks, people that they've mentored, and it allows them to ignore the evidence that Black scientists, especially those who propose to study inequalities in health, not only are less likely to get R01 grants than white scientists, ... but that those Black scientists who do get R01s have higher average review scores than their white counterparts who receive R01s.

I don't know if you've seen the article that came out in January of this year documenting that. That means that their white counterparts are actually assisted in review sections and by NIH directors IN getting grant awards if their proposals don't score at the top of the heap, and it allows them to overlook the finding that of one study that Black scientists report being pushed off the research track by grant review experiences and by a chilly environment among their colleagues and in their universities. So I just give this as an example of how structural racism is embedded in biomedical sciences and how scientists are selected and funded and supported.

And one of the master narratives of the cause of racial inequalities – that's something we explored very well in this series – has been that susceptible individuals have deficient biologies or negative learned behaviors, and that on the population level, some racial "others" are deficient due to *cultures of poverty*, like bad habits that they learn in their families or neighborhoods, or inherited traits – so genetic determinism was another idea that we took on in this series. But I want to emphasize that if we're going to take on research and structural racism and how to address structural racism in our biomedical research, we have to take on the institution of biomedical research itself. And we have an opportunity this year to change that master narrative. I think all of us have been speaking to that, and it's been beautifully explained by my co-panelists.

I just want to leave us with the thought that if we're going to change this system which is a closed loop, it's a very closed loop. So those people who are, consciously are not, a product of a systemically racist biomedical research system, they are in charge of reproducing that system. So we would have to bring people from outside of that system in if we want to make a big change in that loop.

From where I sit, that involves a few things. It certainly involves bringing in scientists who are people of color, who may or may not be in the NIH network, that may be working outside of that, and getting their support elsewhere to making decisions about grants, about promotions, about mentoring. It also, from my point of view, involves bringing in leaders and representatives of affected communities. So I want to endorse a new model of biomedical research that involves community partnership, and I know that many people have been a part of these discussions already do that. But we can amplify that even more. And then I want to leave us with the thought about the biosocial that Hal, I believe, introduced, that we really have to invest significantly more in social and systemic research guided by people with critical perspectives based on their training. For example, in fields that have methods and theories to study systemic racism (sociology, anthropology, political science, economics) and also people with lived experience, people from the affected communities and who have the conditions that we're studying. So, we need a new paradigm of biomedical research that actually amplifies the social part of biosocial processes, like the impact on bodies of systemic racism.

KIRSTEN BIBBINS-DOMINGO: Thank you so much, Helena and Hal. A really terrific way of grounding us in what work we have to do in really transforming our research enterprise. I want to quickly turn to the folks who lead our clinical group, Kevin Grumbach, Malcolm John, and Denise. And then we'll launch into a little bit more free-flowing discussion on how we actually do this work in the next year. Kevin, would you start us off?

KEVIN GRUMBACH: Sure, be happy to. Thanks, Kirsten, and again I want to just start by expressing my appreciation to all the people who organized this remarkable series of symposium events and all the participants who spoke in these events. I learned so much and came in with some ideas, but really deepened my thinking and challenged me in many ways to think differently about things.

For the clinical group, I want to pick up on Helena's comment about master narrative. And really, I think it will link with some of the comments Helena had just made. So for me, one of the most powerful things was starting with the first session and really deepening my understanding of race as a social construct, because I think that's where this whole symposium really was started and grounded. And then, it shattered the false paradigm of race as some biologic, some genetic construct, and really it being a paradigm that's rooted in the ideology of white supremacy. Once you start to then really go there, to think about race as a social construct, I think then you suddenly confront many other paradigms that we have accepted and not questioned. And one of them, for me and I think in the clinical group, was the primacy of the whole mechanistic biomedical model as our guiding framework for how we approach the care of patients and communities.

And so there were some examples that really brought this home. Let's start with the glomerular filtration rate discussion. This is all about that equation that's going to tell you if the GFR is 33 or 28. And the more you think about it, I think for many of us, you realize we're under this illusion that there's that level of precision in any estimate of GFR and you begin to say, does it really make a difference for prescribing metformin if the GFR is 33 or 28? Is that some fixed cut off if suddenly you hit 30 and you're going to get lactic acid doses from metformin and you're not going to get it at 33? And you just begin to start to step back and realize, we are fixated on this idea that there's some biological property that would make a few differences in GFR and not actually thinking about how much of a difference does that actually make in the in the decisions we're making for these patients, and are there really rules that are *that* scientifically based to say that that level of precision is really necessary for how we approach GFR.

Second example – Valy Fontil, I thought, gave a wonderful presentation about hypertension and the whole issue of calcium channel blockers and ACE inhibitors. And again, there's complete overlapping curves about the response among people who are racially identified in different categories. But from a pragmatic point of view, it doesn't make all that much of a difference. Most people are going to respond to either agent, and as you think about it, we get fixated on is it the right drug which has this very mechanistic like for this person with this. Again race is a biologic kind of symbol that it's about the right drug … whether this medication is going to help this person's blood pressure come down, which is much more about are they able to take that pill every day whichever pill you prescribe. Can they afford it? And so we get caught up *in is there a race-based prescribing* instead of actually the real issues that contribute to disparities in hypertension as well as all the stresses around the experience of racism. So there again, as Helena was just saying, if we took more of a whole bio-psycho-social, policy, population focus, we would start putting our attention to much more important things that are the manifestations of structural racism that contribute to disparities in hypertension and outcomes.

Atherosclerotic cardiovascular disease risk formula. Again, Michelle Albert did a beautiful job and really enlightened me to all of that. And I think likely that race, at least Black race, however defined, seems to have predictive power in who's more likely to have heart attacks or stroke in the next 10 years. But there again, we need to be careful of that input to feel comfortable. I left that conversation that Michelle Albert led saying, yeah this actually does have predictive importance. The question is, what is the output then of that formula which we think of it is prescribe a statin or don't prescribe a statin, as opposed to what are the real issues that make this individual more likely to have a bad cardiovascular outcome in the next decade and that we don't have a pill for racism which is really what's driving those adverse outcomes. To not get trapped into thinking that risk prediction is just a guide for us to think about whether to prescribe a statin. It should be a prompt us to think about how we address this whole person and the factors that are contributing to these disparities.

So we didn't talk about VBAC (vaginal birth after cesarean section), but the same issue comes out there. Race, I think from a probabilistic model, it has a predictive value. The answer there again – does the output of it mean this woman shouldn't then be allowed to get a VBAC if she desires, if that is her preference? Or we need to really understand what interventions we could do to lower this person's risk of having a bad outcome should she wish to proceed with a vaginal birth after cesarean section.

So, I think if we're going to dismantle structural racism in patient care, we're probably going to have to also start to chip away at how much the definition of race as of biological construct is actually deeply embedded in this whole mechanistic biomedical framework that has so driven how we approach things. So, I would say we sort of step back. That's how structural racism is so amplified because there's all these other aspects of how we approach health and health care and patients and communities that I think have distracted us from really getting at the most critical factors that are important for the health of the people we take care of. So I took this, and I think many of our group, as a stimulus to think much more broadly about how we take care of people as whole people and understand the complexity of their lives and the factors that contribute to their health.

KIRSTEN BIBBINS-DOMINGO: Thank you, Kevin. Malcolm?

MALCOLM JOHN: Yes, thank you, Kirsten for the invitation to be part of this panel, and I agree with everyone and support the comments to really thank you and the committee for this amazing series. I attended all but one and saw that one on recording. I learned a lot as well. And this is the downside of going last or after Kevin, who gave a great overview, is that he stole a lot of my thunder there. But I did want to share a few additional comments which jumped out at me during this time.

It was clear that education for clinicians is really essential. Most of us are unaware, certainly not to the same degree as some of our trainees, of the role of race in medicine and how we're conflating race and racism. And I think most of us are unaware how that interplays with clinical algorithms and decision making. Kevin mentioned Valy Fontil's ACE inhibitor presentation, and I think that was like a *aha* moment for me, and it really underscored the need to start to work away from routine use of race in medicine and clinical decision making, particularly when they have untoward effects on care, bias, and other forms of misdirection.

We definitely need a higher threshold for using race in our clinical spaces and medicine in general, and there really is a need for more holistic view of our patients including centering patient narratives, particularly around the social determinants of health. Just referring back to another moment in the series when Eliseo spoke and said he starts his initial interviews with new patients with the social history and reviewing the social determinants of health. That was another *aha* moment for me. We need to develop some guidelines for referring to patients within our clinical spaces on rounds and presentations, really underscoring the need for intentionality when we do use it, understanding why we're using it, how it's being used, what its limitations are. And that came up in terms of one of our overall recommendations.

There's also clear need for funding or developing better ways to measure the effects of racism and social determinants of health. This came from Michelle's moment when she talked about ideal modifying factors, and that race really didn't meet the criteria. So precise measurements on the causal pathway and modifiable but social determinants meet some of those, but we need funding, and it's very easy to get – well it's never easy to get NIH funding – but it's relatively easy to get NIH funding to develop new molecular techniques. You can get an R03 or whatever. But it's not easy to get funding to develop new ways of measuring the effects of racism at least in medicine and its impact, and new ways of measuring social determinants of health. So we really need to rethink how we fund the research that then downstream impacts clinical care and we could talk more of that in the open session.

Another thing I will say that given a lot of the uncertainties, some key things on the individual level we need to stop. Like, slow down when you see race used, just like we do for implicit bias to avoid bias in decision making and thinking. Stop. Think. Do we need race in this clinical algorithm or decision making tool that I'm about to use? Because that guideline for hypertension is a national guideline. Most of us accept it at face value. But Valy showed why that may be a mistake. So if you do think it's important, review the primary data and see for yourself. Look at the curve and assess the patient in front of you.

What came up when Dr. Delgado spoke about the eGFR situation with her end-stage renal disease patients – they have muscle wasting, etc. – some of these calculations aren't even relevant and they weren't even included in those studies. So, stop and look at the patient in front of you and definitely look for alternatives that may be race free. And that 'stop and look at the patient in front of you' really underscores could we be thinking of ways to broaden the training around patient narrative experiences and centering those in our EHR and in our clinical presentations in general on the wards.

From an institutional level we need to do the same thing: be accountable for ensuring the safety, effectiveness, and fairness of clinical algorithms that we're using, or clinical decision making tools that we're using regardless of what the national guidelines are. I think one of the recommendations talks through a series of steps on how to do that. And then more, I wouldn't say pie in the sky, but when we talk about precision medicine of course you go on NIH site and it says it's about the genes, the environments, and the lifestyle. But really, we're assuming all these SNP variations and polygenic protocols encompasses that. But really, shouldn't we be looking at those SNPs in addition to a clear patient narrative wrapped around that? That really changes how we might think of precision medicine because I think most of us just immediately go straight to the molecular techniques. So there's more to say, but I'll stop there for starters. Thank you so much

KIRSTEN BIBBINS-DOMINGO: Thanks, Malcolm. Denise?

DENISE CONNOR: Thank you so much. And just to echo what everyone has said, this has been a really, really productive symposium and I'm really grateful to be a part of it and to have learned so much from so many people. One thing that I that really stood out to me was, I believe it was Dorothy Roberts who asked us to consider: why are we obsessed with race? Like why does it come up so much? And to begin to uncover what that might mean, I think Helena's Hansen's comments just now about the master narrative I think is really relevant to both education and the clinical space and the research space, all three.

In particular, in education, the thing I wanted to pull out is that we want our students to learn how to critically critique both new research and what is known, accepted knowledge and not to just accept things at face value. And this shouldn't be difficult. That's what scientists do. We are about curiosity and getting to the why, rather than accepting information that we're receiving. And I think that's a competency that we want all students to develop so that when they enter practice they can continue to consider those problems and how they get underneath what they're learning and what they're seeing to decide if that is actually rigorous science – if that actually makes sense and it's something that we should do or not do. And I think getting in the habit of that kind of critical view every time race comes up, which I'm hearing in many people's comments, is a key thing that I'm hoping our educational enterprise can really foster.

And the only other thing I wanted to pull up is, certainly faculty development is needed to get our faculty ready to talk to students about these issues. Certainly, our students need this sort of increase in their critical view of things. But also what is relevant to education? I think I've heard a little bit of this, but who has expertise? And when are we bringing those folks into the conversation? So when we think about changing curriculum, when we think about changing faculty development, we're still very much looking internally. How do we begin to partner with people who are impacted by racism and other forms of oppression? How do we bring them into this conversation to help us do this work so we're not just deciding on our own how to change things and then expecting it to have a positive impact in the end? How we get enough perspectives and voices into this conversation that are traditionally excluded is a question that I'm really interested in thinking about as well.

KIRSTEN BIBBINS-DOMINGO: Thank you all so much. I really appreciate the very personal nature of the reflections and the impact on specific insights that each of you had with the speakers and the follow-up conversations. I'd like to push us a little bit on what we do next. I think these discussions have been helpful, but we actually want to move towards transforming our systems and we all work on academic medical campuses where teaching, clinical care, and research are all happening simultaneously and they all intersect. Recognizing that this is complex, I'd love you to each talk about what types of concrete steps could we actually take in the next year? What types of systems do we want to have in place to do that type of questioning? So some of this is what should we do? Take race out of eGFR? But then what types of systems do we put in place to say, how should we be using race in this context, or that leads to that type of questioning that Malcolm suggested or that thoughtful reflection? So in your domains, or across domains, what would you like the researchers to do if you're the educator or the clinicians... what can we do in this next year?

MALCOLM JOHN: I was just going to say to elevate the humanities and social sciences in pairing with us. I think the REPAIR project has started a process that's gained a lot of respect and influencing our thinking in terms of our understanding the history of race in medicine, the origins of some of our leading institutions, and also our role as a health system, what happened here at UCSF in contributing to racial inequities and supporting the white supremacy structure within medicine. I think that that's an essential history and because without understanding history we will make the mistakes over and over again. So I vote for elevating the humanities and social sciences within our health institution as a starting point, but I'm curious because this is the question I have as well. So I'm interested to hear from others.

KIRSTEN BIBBINS-DOMINGO: Great. Catherine, and then Hal?

CATHERINE LUCEY: Yeah, so I vote with Malcolm as usual. But I also vote for us to take a critical lens, the same lens you've used in this series, to all of our important systems with an expectation that we will find, within each of those systems, manifestations of structural racism that need to be uncovered. And I use the four A's. *Admissions*, that is who comes in as a student, a resident, a faculty, a staff person. The system of *assessment*, how do we evaluate their worth and their value and their growth in their positions? *Advancement*, who gets promoted, chosen for leadership positions? And then *accountability*, how do we hold people accountable for appropriate competencies not just in their own discipline but in the core disciplines that make us a community. So those issues of anti-racism and pro-equity.

And I think if we were to take a deep dive into each of these systems and say, in what way does the current way in which we do this either mitigate or reinforce structural racism, I think we would find a lot to work on. And in the end, we can't count on people as individuals to be perfect. We have to be able to surround them with systems that make it easier than not for them to do what we want them to do. So I'd vote for a deep dive into these systems in the next 12 to 18 months, to say we are going to redesign to eliminate any discrimination or bias that is holding people back from either joining our communities, thriving in our communities, or doing the very best they can to solve big problems and take great care of patients.

KIRSTEN BIBBINS-DOMINGO: Thank you. Helena, and then I'll turn to Hal. What I'd love to push each of the speakers on… so we had the broad goals for our institution, but part of the intent of this series was really to focus on how we use racial categorizations. I'd love you to speak to that specifically. Not to say that that is everything. It is not the larger construct. But it there some way in which focusing on that is specific enough to have some specific solutions or specific ways to approach that actually lend to the discussion of the larger challenges of structural racism within our institution. But I'd love us to get specific. I don't know who was next, Hal or Helena, and then Kevin?

HAL COLLARD: So, Kirsten, you moved the goal post a little bit there. But that's good. I like the idea of being specific, and maybe this comment relates to both, but I want to pick up on a couple of terrific comments by our panelists. I think that we want to change the core narrative, and I love Malcolm's focus on stopping and thinking and recognizing that there's an important question here around race and racism in what we're doing so. And then I think Catherine's point about a structural solution… I feel like there are structural tools, ways in which we can as an institution enable facilitate, incentivize this important conversation and reflection. So one thing that I think has been – just trying to think practically – very useful for me is the PRIDE values.

If I think about things that are across mission and ways in which we've tried to integrate a conversation in a way that highlights some of the key aspects that are important to that conversation, I feel like the focus on the PRIDE values at the UC's – and I don't know if that's a UCSF specific initiative or across UC – but it's an acronym. And I think that we could consider something similar for this, and that could apply both to the broader issues [of] foundational structural racism underlying the many manifestations of that, or more specifically to the issue you just posed, Kirsten, around how we address race specifically in clinical care, research, and education. I just wanted to float that as an idea for a short-term approach that delivers a tangible focused institutional structural tool to help us all be aware of stop and think and work to change the narrative here

KIRSTEN BIBBINS-DOMINGO: Great. Helena, and then Kevin.

HELENA HANSEN: I appreciate your request that we focus and be concrete, so I'm going to try to be. I don't think, though, that we can separate the way that we use racial categories from how our systems are set up, so my comments will always come back to that. And I think I'm echoing pretty much all of my co-panelists here in thinking about systemic change. That's really what our discussions have been crying out for.

And so just thinking very concretely about how we can affect systemic change so that the racial categorizations, the way that we use them, actually lead back to systemic change – we have to begin with the systems that we are embedded in, and imagining how concretely that would work. So those bodies that set the agenda and determine support, money, other kinds of institutional support for activity. So let's take research, let's take review sections, or let's say take promotion review bodies – they have to have a different composition because as Catherine Lucey was explaining, we can't leave this up to well-intentioned individuals. This is really a systemic issue and so we have to proactively demand that any review body that allocates research funding or decides on hiring or promotion of researchers (and this applies, I think, to education and clinical work as well) that those review bodies proactively include people of color, they include members of affected communities. That's very, very important and we have colleagues, for example, who work with tribal leaders in Native American communities that do that, where tribal leaders are part of the review process.

AIDS activism showed us how that works as well. The very idea that people who are HIV positive or directly affected by HIV, sitting on scientific review sections at NIH, sitting on Ryan White Care Act, health care many allocation bodies – that's a model that we should weave throughout. As well as social scientists. I'm really very gratified that my co-panelists have identified social scientists, humanities scholars as people who should be more integrally involved. So that also means sitting in decision-making bodies.

We could also look proactively to, for example, funders that have taken a different, less narrow, much more social determinant, structural racism approach to research on inequalities. One of them that I'm familiar with is Robert Wood Johnson Foundation, where their Cultures Of Health initiative has really restructured the way that they develop grant requests for proposals, review proposals, and set a scientific agenda. So I think we should look to those kinds of funders and institutions for models of how to retool our allocation of resources.

And when I say we, that could be UC system as a start, and hopefully spreading to other academic medical centers. And then I want to hold up HBCUs. Many of you are maybe familiar with the statistic that historically Black colleges and universities produce 70 [percent] of the nation's [African American] doctors, and they're a pretty small set of institutions. That's profound. They're often disparaged as somehow not as good as predominantly white institutions. I want to argue that they are centers of excellence that we need to study and proactively borrow and adapt techniques from. They're doing something right. They have got right in what they are doing. We do sadly very poorly compared to them in terms of – I mean predominantly white institutions – producing scientists and clinical practitioners, physicians of color. And so I would say proactively study and partner with them so that we can do a better job.

And then lastly, look to other countries. So we are a country that spends the most per capita of any country in the world on healthcare and we have the worst outcomes of any industrialized nation. Many of that statistic. A lot of it is due to structural racism. I'm not saying structural racism doesn't exist in other countries, including Canada, France, etc., but we have a tremendous amount to learn from them in terms of how they structure their healthcare systems and their research agendas. And so I would say we should look beyond our borders as well. But if we could just begin by looking at HBCUs – they are doing something that actively redresses structural racism in research, clinical work, and in education, and we should learn from that.

KIRSTEN BIBBINS-DOMINGO: Great. I'm going to keep pushing you all to be a little bit concrete on this, and I think Kevin is probably up next. When I think about Kevin and Malcolm, both of you have been involved in our health equity council at UCSF. One of the major initiatives of the health equity council at UCSF health was actually to make sure that that field, self-identified race, was not left blank in for our patients. So that means when you come in as a patient at UCSF health, we're going to ask you that question. We think it's important for your care. Why do we think it's important for your care? How do you reconcile that or how do you explain that to people? Because I know each of you have been in these discussions. Well, why is it important that we do this at UCSF health? And why, if we've gone through this trouble of measuring this, why did we take the Black race out of the eGFR equation? So, help us to understand. We are using this. In fact, we doubled down on measuring this. So what does that mean? Kevin or Malcolm?

MALCOLM JOHN: I was coming up with a list of concrete actions as well. But I think Kirsten's point is well taken. While we exist in this current reality, it is important to look for disparities and to ask the question of why they exist and how to address them. And in fact, one of the recommendations from the subgroup at the previous gathering was to actually broaden the race/ethnicity categories for more inclusive and nuanced representation even if they have to be rolled up into more meaningful variables later for health equity analyses.

So I think it's important that people understand that focused context. Again, it's not that we cannot use race until we get to a better system. It is just having intentionality and a higher threshold for when we use it and being very clear on the purpose and utility of it. And I think for the sake of identifying health care disparities, which is right in our wheelhouse – things around access, experience, and outcomes – we must do that today. That is just an area. But that is different than applying race in clinical algorithms and clinical decision making and the way we use that language on the clinical wards in describing patients and having an implication of what that means when I say a Black woman comes yelling in the ER, was loud in the ER, etc. So, I think I will lean on our colleague Alicia Fernandez who always says in these areas, it's important to be more nuanced and flexible and really look at the use case very carefully, individual case by case, and be clear on the intent. And I would say that that's probably why we recommended this. But I have some other concrete recommendations but I want to give the floor to Kevin because he was ahead of me.

KIRSTEN BIBBINS-DOMINGO: Yeah, I just want to react to that for a second and just say I agree. And I guess the question is, we have measured this and we have talked about the challenges of having that measurement in our systems because we use them for all sorts of things. So how then do we create the structures to enable people to understand when might one use this concept? When is it not appropriate? When do we not know? How do we become more fluent in our way of talking about and thinking about this? One of the big critiques throughout this has been we don't want to be in a color-blind, race-blind society. That means in our campuses, we have to be in a way where people can understand what its use means in a particular....

MALCOLM JOHN: Yeah. That's a great point and I think two things. Around healthcare and the health equity space, we are being led by Sarah Lahidji, our program manager and future director of health equity, in developing a toolkit to help clinical units understand how to use this information, how to apply in a way that does not promote more disparities, etc. So I think a toolkit that is being developed by the department of quality and safety is essential on the clinical side. One of the recommendations from our last session is to develop a toolkit for how to use race on the wards and guide people through that and how to apply it in patient narratives if at all. So I think one of the concrete recommendations that I feel is important is developing guidelines and a toolkit on when to use race in the ward, how to use it in presentations, how to assess any clinical guideline or algorithm that actually uses race, that sort of 'stop, think, look' etc. And whenever you go to use race, whether in a clinical guideline algorithm, on the wards, or in your disparities improvement work, why are you using race? How are you measuring it? How are you interpreting? And the lesson I learned from Valy's presentation is, how is that information presented?

Sometimes you will have some negative impact even when you're trying to achieve a more positive impact in the short term. So identify that and identify how will you ameliorate it. But again, I think Helena is right. We're trying to work within our current broken framework and we really need to think more broadly. And she reminded me that, and Hal of course knows this, the office of research anti-racism task force is going to be coming out with some recommendations. And many of the things Helena recommended – I was on the infrastructure subcommittee – we are talking about and hopefully will show up in our final recommendations, including increasing partnerships with HBCUs. So I got off a little bit on topic at the end there, but I hope that answered your question, Kirsten.

KIRSTEN BIBBINS-DOMINGO: Yeah, so let me probe a little bit more. So part of the reason I was really motivated for this discussion is because we have outstanding scholars on our campus who have differences of opinion on this topic and who will draw on bodies of evidence and come to different conclusions. What's the way in which we can continue to create environments that both allow for nuanced discussion, but also push us to action at the same time, because we also have to continue to transform our system. So what are the ways that we do that? Anyone want to… I can't tell whose hands are up or everyone's ignoring me now. Hal?

TAKESHA COOPER: Okay. Yeah, for some reason I don't have the option to raise my hand, so I I've been letting people know I have something to say. So I wanted to think about specifics in particular, and I think we really have to go back and really reify that racism as a social construct. We have to get people comfortable talking about race, and our entire nation has problems discussing race. But as physicians, as researchers, we have a responsibility to our patients to delve deeply into how race impacts on the health of our patients.

I think we on this panel are quite open to the discussion, but I can imagine at your institutions many of your colleagues are not comfortable having these conversations and would rather avoid the topic I think altogether. So more conversations I think is what we need. Discussing the impacts of racism in our faculty meetings, journal clubs, grand rounds, maybe having mandatory reading for all medical students, *Medical Apartheid*, *Fatal Invention* by Dorothy Roberts, and then having ongoing discussions afterwards. Maybe requiring, in order for admission to medical school, we ask for biology, o-chem, physics, math, but what if we required all students to take a course on critical race theory? That way we're already bringing in students who've had some of this background and that we can expand on it when they're in medical school. I think that's really important. I think only once, when we're able to fully have deep conversations about race, then we can begin to more universally consider how race and medicine impacts our patients, impacts our care of our patients. So, thanks.

KIRSTEN BIBBINS-DOMINGO: Terrific, Takesha. I really appreciate your comments. Who's next, since I totally blown it as a moderator.

DENISE CONNOR: Can I just add onto that? I really appreciated those comments, Takesha, and I would just add that we have to be thoughtful about white supremacy culture and the ways that it gets into our way of addressing racism. So of course there's urgency to address racism. There's been urgency for, what, 200 plus years in this country. But if we are so focused on the check boxes and what are we going to do now, without allowing inclusivity and full discussion and honoring the process as well as the end point, we're not going to get anywhere. So we're not going to solve racism in the next year.

I think we need to just be able to turn down the volume a little of how we've always done things and think about is there a new paradigm for how to do this work. I think as Malcolm John pointed out, looking to our social science colleagues to learn from them a little bit about that and to get out of this sort of very goal-oriented way that we do things in in biomedical world is one important thing, and it kind of comes back to what Takesha just said, which is conversations themselves are an end point. Getting comfortable having conversations or being uncomfortable sitting with discomfort is itself a very valuable and important outcome. We might not be able to say, look now we have a number we can point to to say that we've sort of achieved a goal, but that process itself should be highly valued. And inclusivity and who is being brought into this conversation and who has the space and the time to be heard is equally valid and important. So, I think that's one other thing I would just sort of add to the great comments already.

CATHERINE LUCEY: I'll jump in. I just want to give a very specific example of what we could accomplish, going back to what Kirsten had challenged us with. And I really appreciate the call for greater conversations that are informed, not just opinion driven. So informed with evidence from multiple different disciplines. But here's an example of where we might think about a systemic change that could happen if we put our minds to it, probably in 12 to 18 months, and that is our electronic health records.

Malcolm talked very wisely about the importance of changing the way we think about race in our clinical presentations. I'm going to argue that we need to think about race and how we deal with it from the very beginning of the patient encounter, and we could restructure our electronic health record, the problem-oriented medical record, to not be a problem-oriented medical record, but to be a patient health record that enables us to use race as an asset.

Race/ethnicity, gender identity as an asset element, rather than pathologize race which is what we typically do when we say this is a Black person and we know Black people are more likely to get glaucoma. We never say white people are more likely to get cataracts. We pathologize race in a way that's not helpful. We should really think about restructuring the problem-oriented medical record to reflect our contemporary understanding of race and racism and to get rid of things that are structurally discriminating.

We talk about lifestyle choices, and when our social history is confined to 'do you drink' and 'do you smoke' as if those are the only relevant social history, we're already buying into to what I think will be the take-home message of the day, the master narrative, that actually people have a choice about some of the things that they are subjected to in the social aspects of their lives whether it's poverty, experiencing homelessness, substance use disorders, or things like that. So we could really think about redesigning the problem-oriented medical record to being a patient care record or patient health record that both celebrates the real assets of their community, their culture, their ethnicity and also honors the experiences that they've endured *en route* to the medical environment and think a little bit about what Michelle Albert had talked about, which is what are truly modifying factors that we could engage with.

And so we can't expect that every single person knows how to do that on their own as they're thrust into the clinical environment. But with the largest system we use in the healthcare environment, the electronic health record, we could redesign how data is collected, how people view these elements, and we could really make I think a broader synergistic change not only for medical students but also for residents, and faculty nurses, and even clerks who are engaging with information that's collected and codified in that record.

KIRSTEN BIBBINS-DOMINGO: Yeah, it's a great suggestion because it's also a backbone that spans across the different domains that we're talking about in the end in lots of ways. Hal and then Helena?

HAL COLLARD: Yeah so I'll try to be quick here. I just want to thank, by the way, the listeners for some of the questions in the Q&A. They're terrific and I hope we capture them and address them at some point down the line. Yeah, Kirsten I wanted to respond directly to your question about how we move this difficult, challenging issue forward. Takesha and Denise's comments really resonated with me, too. And I think I was going to make a similar point about not pressing too quickly for answers and check boxes, but also recognizing that that's very unsatisfying to a lot of people who appropriately, all of us, really want change now and want to make some concrete interventions.

I want to suggest that the solution going forward is very much what you've developed here, Kirsten. It's a space for listening, discussion, debate that is respectful, that's welcoming, that's multi stakeholder and multi-dimensional, and that identifies and isn't afraid then to test and reflect on specific ideas that may make a difference in moving the larger vision forward. So, I think – and this is an evidence-based suggestion – difficult problems are best solved by groups. That is a fact, so I think that taking a collective view of this is the right way to go and we should identify what the priorities are out of these groups and as an institution commit to testing them, but bringing them back to this as the foundation of moving forward – a continued conversation. I want to just point out one other quick comment which is there are research approaches to dealing with these types of issues, when there's an absence of traditional objective data. There are Delphi methodologies, there are other methodologies that are designed specifically to help come to some consensus prioritization of shared views around difficult issues where you we feel like again we lack at traditional sources of evidence. So we might consider that as one strategy out of this more foundational conversation we're having. But you had asked us this question ahead of time, Kirsten, and I thought a lot about the way to address complex and thorny topics, and I really think you're on to it here. If we can find a way to keep people engaged and keep this conversation going as a community, that will spin off a lot of very useful and impactful change.

KIRSTEN BIBBINS-DOMINGO: Thanks, Hal. I have to say, I appreciated your comment at the beginning. I do think that we've brought many more people into this and I think some of this is it is skill building amongst people who are not thinking about this topic all the time but want to approach it in the right way in their research question. There are ways to connect and I think the points that Helena has made repeatedly about our social scientists, the perspectives that they bring, that are really important to think of this across disciplines, I think a consultation like the CTSI has used for years but focused on this topic I think can help many, many more people to have the skills to at least understand how to approach this topic. Helena and then Malcolm? We only have four minutes, so I urge you to keep your comments brief.

HELENA HANSEN: Okay, thank you. Well I appreciate the full range of suggestions here that are ranging from really concrete first steps that we can make, conversations to have, things to add to the electronic medical record, to more substantial systemic change which I think Denise most recently brought up. I just want to say I have a fear. I have a fear that the conversation we're having today, even though it's hopeful and forward thinking, that it could be a flash in the pan if it is limited to the conversations and kind of consciousness building that we've been discussing. I think we definitely have to track who's making decisions in biomedicine and where the money is going. We just have to do that. And it has to be tied directly to the conceptual frameworks.

How do we understand the importance of that? But we have we critically have to put people who are affected directly by the health inequalities that bring us to the table now at the decision-making table and in charge of funds allocation. And so we have to track that. It cannot simply be conversations, because these are difficult conversations for a reason. They involve power. They involve resources. We're in a society that really punishes those that don't have access to power, and it's scary for people who have power to think about losing it. We have a moment in which there's some political organizing and some political will to at least open up conversations like this, and if we don't take it all the way to really attend to who's making decisions, where money is going in a substantial way, we will lose this window of opportunity. It will be it will be limited to the kind of low-hanging fruit of let's put a question in the EMR, have conversations with people who are already at the table, as opposed to the universe of the people who are not at the table. And that's the crux of the problem.

MALCOLM JOHN: I just wanted to follow up with what both Helena and Hal said. I really support the idea of continuing this dialogue because we're just getting started. There's a need to collect some baseline data or cataloging of how we're currently using race in medicine in our different spaces (education, clinical, and research) and we need to have a way of monitoring the impact of changes, such as the eGFR changes we've made. It may not come out of this group, the monitoring work, but it could be through collaborative process sort of like we do with the health equity council. So working with the health equity council or other groups. I think it's really important, as Hal said, to bring in this multi-disciplinary clinical folks, educational folks, clinical researchers, social scientists, basic scientists. I didn't reference the things we learned about from pharmacogenomics and other benefits and really how this can change the care to be really more patient-centered way of precision medicine in a really redefined way and trauma-informed way as well. So I want to second what Hal said, and of course what Helena said. Thank you.

KIRSTEN BIBBINS-DOMINGO: Thank you, Malcolm. So we are at the end of our time, sadly. People are already asking whether the transcript of this discussion will be available, and it will. In fact, we're working on putting a transcript together of the entire symposium for people not interested in watching YouTube videos and would rather want to see it in written form. We also are trying to think of other ways to disseminate shorter aspects of this.

I think a lot of really important ideas have been generated and mostly the platform for having these discussions have been important. We had a great conversation with the Robert Wood Johnson Foundation yesterday to talk about what does it mean to continue to have these conversations so that in our enterprises (academic medical centers), we're actually moving forward in concrete ways. And I really thank you all for engaging in this work and for being part of this final discussion, but mostly for being really committed. And it's all on record today to continue to advance the discussion going forward in the next year across our campuses and look forward to working with all of you in this work as well as all of you who have participated in these sessions as a part of the audience, contributing great questions and sparking the follow-up conversations. We're going to need many people to be part of this really important critical conversation for transforming our institution. It'll involve all of us in this work.

So, thank you again for being a part.

www.ingramcontent.com/pod-product-compliance
Lightning Source LLC
LaVergne TN
LVHW022207200926
848481LV00006B/1876
* 9 7 8 1 7 3 5 5 4 2 3 4 8 *